Workbook for Hartman's Complete Guide for the Medication Aide

SECOND EDITION

Hartman Publishing, Inc.

hartmanonline.com

Hartman

Credits

Managing Editor
Susan Alvare Hedman

Developmental Editor
Kristin Calderon

Cover Designer
Kirsten Browne

Cover Illustrator
Iveta Vaicule

Production
Tracy Kopsachilis

Proofreaders
Zella Mansson
Rachel Scott

Copyright Information

1313 Iron Ave SW
Albuquerque, New Mexico 87102
(505) 291-1274
web: hartmanonline.com
email: orders@hartmanpublishing.com

ISBN 978-1-60425-179-1

PRINTED IN THE USA

Notice to Readers

Though the guidelines and procedures contained in this text are based on consultations with healthcare professionals, they should not be considered absolute recommendations. The instructor and readers should follow employer, local, state, and federal guidelines concerning healthcare practices. These guidelines change, and it is the reader's responsibility to be aware of these changes and of the policies and procedures of their healthcare facility.

The publisher, author, editors, and reviewers cannot accept any responsibility for errors or omissions or for any consequences from application of the information in this book and make no warranty, express or implied, with respect to the contents of the book. The publisher does not warrant or guarantee any of the products described herein or perform any analysis in connection with any of the product information contained herein.

Gender Usage

This workbook uses gender pronouns interchangeably to denote healthcare team members and residents. The words *male* and *female* as used throughout relate to a person's sex assigned at birth. This may be different from their experienced gender.

Table of Contents

Preface iv

1 The Medication Aide in Healthcare Settings 1

2 Ethical and Legal Issues 5

3 Medication Basics 11

4 Medication Orders and Documentation 17

5 Medication Dosage 21

6 Medication Side Effects, Reactions, and Interactions 23

7 Medication Safety 27

8 Preparation and Administration of Medication 31

9 Preventing and Responding to Medication Errors 41

10 The Integumentary System and Common Medications 45

11 The Musculoskeletal System and Common Medications 49

12 The Nervous System and Common Medications 53

13 The Circulatory System and Common Medications 59

14 The Respiratory System and Common Medications 63

15 The Urinary System and Common Medications 67

16 The Gastrointestinal System and Common Medications 71

17 The Endocrine System and Common Medications 77

18 The Reproductive System and Common Medications 79

19 The Immune and Lymphatic Systems and Common Medications 81

Procedure Checklists 85

Practice Exam 97

Preface

Welcome to the *Workbook for Hartman's Complete Guide for the Medication Aide*! This workbook is designed to help you review what you have learned from reading your textbook. For this reason, the workbook is organized around learning objectives, just like the textbook and your instructor's teaching material.

These learning objectives work as a built-in study guide. After completing the exercises for each learning objective in the workbook, ask yourself if you can DO what that learning objective describes.

If you can, move on to the next learning objective. If you cannot, just go back to the textbook, reread that learning objective, and try again.

We have provided procedure checklists at the end of the workbook. There is also a final exam that can serve as practice if your state has a certification exam. The answers to the workbook exercises and the exam are in your instructor's teaching guide.

Happy learning!

1

The Medication Aide in Healthcare Settings

1. Describe the medication aide's role

Multiple Choice

Circle the letter of the answer that best completes the statement or answers the question.

1. Who supervises unlicensed healthcare workers such as nursing assistants and medication aides?
   (A) More experienced unlicensed healthcare workers
   (B) Facility administrators
   (C) Facility owners
   (D) Licensed professionals such as nurses or doctors

2. In addition to long-term care facilities, in which of the following types of facilities do some states allow MAs to work?
   (A) Urgent care centers
   (B) Standalone emergency rooms
   (C) Group homes for people with intellectual disabilities
   (D) Public schools

3. Which of these tasks is commonly allowed for MAs?
   (A) Deciding when to give residents an over-the-counter medication
   (B) Giving oral medications ordered by a provider to medically stable residents
   (C) Adjusting a resident's insulin dosage based on blood sugar levels
   (D) Suggesting changes to a resident's medications based on observations of the resident's condition

4. In some states an MA may be called
   (A) Pharmacy technician
   (B) Medication technician
   (C) Medical assistant
   (D) Patient care technician

5. In most states an MA is not allowed to
   (A) Give a resident a new medication the first time the resident takes it
   (B) Give a resident food to go with a medication that must be taken with food
   (C) Measure a resident's vital signs
   (D) Observe a resident for any changes or possible effects from a medication

2. Discuss professionalism and list examples of professional behavior

Short Answer

For each of the items below, write P *for professional or* NP *for not professional.*

1. ____ Checking social media accounts while waiting for a resident to swallow medications
2. ____ Accepting a gift card given by a resident's daughter during the holidays
3. ____ Calling the facility first thing in the morning to report an illness that will prevent the MA from working that day
4. ____ Reporting right away if a resident refuses to take a medication
5. ____ Teasingly calling a resident "my girlfriend"
6. ____ Washing hands less often when there are no cases of contagious illnesses going around the facility

Short Answer

7. List one situation in which an MA should *not* accept a delegated task.

____

____

____

8. Give an example of how an MA can be *conscientious* on the job.

____

____

____

9. How does working professionally as a team help healthcare workers protect patient safety?

____

____

____

____

3. Discuss chain of command and scope of practice

True or False

Mark each statement with either a T *for true or an* F *for false.*

1. ____ In the chain of command, an MA is below the provider who prescribes a medication and above the nurse who provides daily care for the resident.
2. ____ The chain of command exists only to protect MAs and their employers from liability.
3. ____ Scope of practice defines the tasks that healthcare workers are allowed to do based on state laws and facility policies.
4. ____ It is acceptable for an MA to do a task outside their scope of practice if it is assigned and directly supervised by a doctor.
5. ____ Each state grants the right to practice medical professions such as nursing and medicine.
6. ____ If a resident has a bad reaction to a medication that an MA administers, the MA is legally responsible for any harm even if they were following facility policy and administering the drug under the supervision of a nurse.
7. ____ It is beyond an MA's scope of practice to discuss diagnosis and treatment plans with a resident or resident's family.
8. ____ In some states/facilities, an MA may not be allowed to perform routine care tasks that do not relate to medications even if they were trained as a nursing assistant and used to provide that care.

Matching

For each of the numbered items, write the letter that best matches the term. Use each letter only once.

9. ____ Assessment
10. ____ Diagnosis
11. ____ Evaluation
12. ____ Implementation
13. ____ Nursing process
14. ____ Planning

(A) Putting a care plan into action; giving care

(B) The communication process that allows team members to provide for a resident's care needs on an ongoing basis

(C) Identifying health problems

(D) Getting information from many sources and reviewing this information to identify actual or potential problems

(E) Examining carefully to see whether goals have been met or progress achieved

(F) Setting goals and creating a care plan to meet the resident's needs

4. Discuss communication, team building, and interpersonal relationships

Short Answer

1. List three types of people MAs must communicate with regularly.

____

____

____

2. What is the three-step process that repeats over and over during a conversation?

____

____

____

3. How can the same words spoken in a different way communicate a different message?

____

____

____

____

4. A resident has just returned from the hospital, where surgery to remove cancer was not completely successful. How can an MA respond in a way that does not use a cliché? Give an example.

____

____

____

5. An MA is administering medications to a resident who had been having nausea after taking an antibiotic. The MA asks, "Is your tummy better now?" How could the MA ask about the nausea and get more information? Give an example.

____

____

____

6. What is wrong with this statement from an MA to a resident? "It doesn't say this on the label, but I'll bet your nausea is from having dairy products with the medication. You should stop drinking milk or eating yogurt while you're taking it."

____

____

____

Fill in the Blank

7. Active listening means focusing on the person _______________ the message and giving _______________.

8. Using _______________ for a few moments at a time allows the resident to think about what to say.

9. The MA should respect residents' religious _______________, practices, or lack of _______________.

10. The MA should _______________ _______________ before touching residents and should respect their preferences.

11. The MA should make sure _______________ _______________ are clean and in proper working order. These include hearing aids, eyeglasses, dentures, and wrist or hand braces.

12. Because medications can cause changes in health and behavior that may be cause for concern, good communication with residents promotes _______________.

Short Answer

For each of the following statements, write Y *if it may help resolve conflict and* N *if it is not likely to help resolve conflict.*

13. _____ Allow your emotions to control how you respond to a situation that is causing conflict.

14. _____ Make sure body language is not threatening.

15. _____ Use a conversation about one situation as a way to discuss other problems you have had with the same person in the past.

16. _____ Use sarcasm to emphasize your points.

17. _____ Address conflict early on, before bad feelings grow.

18. _____ Be prepared to compromise.

19. _____ Discuss the situation in a public place to make sure everyone remains calm.

5. Explain policy and procedure manuals

Multiple Choice

1. In a healthcare facility, a policy
   (A) Is a course of action that should be taken every time a certain situation occurs
   (B) Is a method, or way, of doing something
   (C) Is a law passed by the federal government that applies to the facility
   (D) Is an optional guide that suggests good ways to manage common situations

2. Which of these is a common policy at long-term care facilities?
   (A) MAs use souffle cups (small disposable cups) when preparing a resident's medications
   (B) MAs must pass a certification test
   (C) MAs must only perform tasks assigned to them
   (D) MAs can choose to continue NA care tasks if they like, whether or not they are assigned to do so

3. The requirement to keep resident information confidential
   (A) Is one that may vary by facility
   (B) Relates only to medical diagnoses
   (C) Does not apply when the MA is speaking to a family member
   (D) Is both a facility policy and a law

4. Which of the following is true?
   (A) An MA should never skip any of the steps in a procedure for administering a medication.
   (B) An MA can skip identification steps after they get to know the residents they give medications to.
   (C) An MA can skip steps related to checking things like medication name, dose, and time after they have administered a specific medication to the same resident at least two times before.
   (D) An MA can skip steps about removing or avoiding distractions after 3 months on the job without errors.

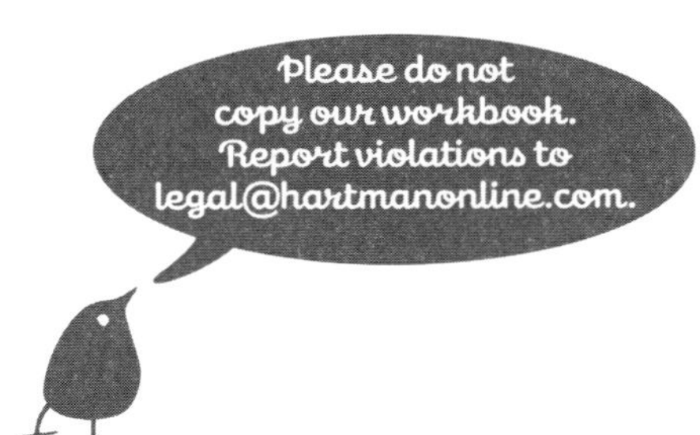

2

Ethical and Legal Issues

1. Describe legal and ethical behavior for medication aides

Short Answer

For each of the following examples, decide whether the issue is a legal or an ethical issue. Write L *for legal or* E *for ethical.*

1. _____ When Maria is at home with her husband she makes fun of the way a resident she gives medications to speaks English.

2. _____ A resident's granddaughter gave her an older cell phone that the resident never learned to use. Dennis takes the phone while the resident is using the bathroom and gives it to a friend.

3. _____ Imani is 15 minutes late coming in for work on Monday. Her supervisor does not notice, and Imani does not tell her.

4. _____ Rachel is excited to see that the grandmother of a well-known musician is a new resident at the facility where she works. She takes a picture of the musician visiting her grandmother and sends it to her friends.

5. _____ Alex works in a state where MAs are not allowed to administer controlled medications. He is in a resident's room when the nurse gives the resident an opioid painkiller and the resident drops it. Alex pretends to help the nurse find the pill, but instead puts it in his pocket to sell to a friend.

Read the scenarios below and then answer the questions that follow.

Sarah, an MA at a long-term care facility, is out shopping with her friends. One of them asks her if she likes her job, and she responds enthusiastically. She then tells them about Mrs. Calvert, who hates taking medications and makes faces every time Sarah brings them to her. She shows them pictures she has taken of Mrs. Calvert's expressions.

6. Did Sarah behave in a legal and ethical manner? Why or why not?

____

____

____

____

____

Mr. Shelton, a resident Sarah cares for, requests Tylenol for a headache. The nurse approves the medication and assigns Sarah to administer it. After Mr. Shelton takes the medication Sarah realizes that she administered a higher dose than what is listed on Mr. Shelton's medication administration record. Because Tylenol is an over-the-counter medication and Mr. Shelton is generally healthy, Sarah does not report her mistake. She documents having given him the correct dose.

7. Did Sarah behave in a legal and ethical manner? Why or why not?

____

____

____

____

____

2. Discuss how state laws affect the role of medication aides

Short Answer

Make a check mark (✓) next to parts of an MA's job that are likely to be defined by state law.

1. ____ The hours an MA is assigned to work
2. ____ What types of medications an MA is allowed to administer
3. ____ What types of facilities can employ an MA
4. ____ Whether an MA must wear scrubs of a particular color
5. ____ The type of training an MA receives before administering medications
6. ____ Whether an MA must take a certification exam
7. ____ Whether MAs work alone or in pairs
8. ____ What type of documentation (paper or electronic) the MA uses
9. ____ Whether an MA must first be certified and have experience as a nursing assistant

Fill in the Blank

10. MAs are allowed to administer certain types of medications, such as those given by ____________________, those applied to a body surface, and those placed in the ear, eye, or nose. Many states do not allow MAs to give residents medications that are considered ____________________ substances.
11. All states require that MAs provide medications only under the supervision of a ____________________ or other ____________________ healthcare professional.
12. States vary on rules about giving medications by certain routes, such as ____________________, which uses a machine that allows a patient to breathe in a medicated mist.
13. If a nurse or provider requests that an MA perform a task they are not trained to perform, the MA must ____________________.

3. Explain tasks that cannot be delegated to medication aides

Multiple Choice

1. Converting a medication dose means
   (A) Calculating how much of a generic medication such as ibuprofen to substitute for a name brand medication such as Advil
   (B) Calculating how much of an over-the-counter medication to substitute for a prescription medication
   (C) Making a change from one measurement system to another
   (D) Adjusting a dose based on the weight of the patient
2. Which of the following healthcare workers is allowed to assess a patient's need for a PRN medication?
   (A) A nursing assistant
   (B) A nurse
   (C) A medication aide
   (D) A facility's activities director
3. Most states do not allow MAs to administer
   (A) Over-the-counter medications
   (B) Injected medications
   (C) Blood pressure medications
   (D) Antibiotics
4. Copying information from a prescription into a resident's medical record, or ____________________ a medication order, is beyond the scope of practice for an MA.
   (A) Receiving
   (B) Confirming
   (C) Transcribing
   (D) Finalizing

5. MAs are usually not allowed to administer a(n) __________________ medication for the __________________ time.
   (A) New, first
   (B) Strong, first
   (C) Heart, final
   (D) Diabetes, meal

6. This type of injection is used to administer insulin to residents with diabetes and is allowed for MAs in a limited number of states:
   (A) Intravenous
   (B) Subcutaneous
   (C) Intramuscular
   (D) Intradermal

7. Which of these tasks may MAs be allowed to do in some states?
   (A) Insert a feeding tube
   (B) Irrigate a feeding tube (flush it out with saline)
   (C) Remove a feeding tube
   (D) Administer medications through a feeding tube

8. In some states MAs may be trained and allowed to test blood sugar (glucose) in this way:
   (A) By drawing blood from the inner elbow
   (B) By finger stick
   (C) By collecting a saliva specimen
   (D) By testing a stool specimen

4. Discuss the medication aide's role in delegated tasks

Short Answer

For each of the following examples, decide whether the question about delegation must be answered by the nurse or by the MA. Write N *for nurse or* M *for MA.*

1. _____ Can I be available to give supervision and support?
2. _____ What is the level of resident stability?
3. _____ Does this task fall within my scope of practice?
4. _____ Can I give appropriate direction and communication?
5. _____ Do I have the necessary skills to do this task?
6. _____ Do my supervisor and I both understand who is doing what?
7. _____ Is there a match between the resident's needs and the skills, abilities, and experience of the person this task is delegated to?
8. _____ Do I have all the information I need to do this job?

Fill in the Blank

9. If the MA feels she does not have the __________________ for a task or that the task is not within her __________________ __________________ __________________, she should not complete the task and should talk to the nurse.

10. Having been delegated a task for one resident does not mean the MA can perform this task for __________________ __________________.

11. Although it may be difficult for an MA to refuse a task for which they are not trained or that is beyond their scope of practice, resident __________________, the law, and __________________ all require that the MA refuse.

5. Explain Residents' Rights and describe person-centered care

True or False

1. _____ Residents waive (give up) their rights to make independent choices when they move into an LTCF.
2. _____ Residents must be given a written copy of their rights in a language they can understand.
3. _____ If a resident speaks a language that is not common in the area where the LTCF is located, the resident and/or family members must provide their own interpretation services.

4. ____ Moving into an LTCF means agreeing to appear in social media posts promoting the facility and in photos on the facility's website.

5. ____ Residents must be treated with dignity and respect by caregivers.

6. ____ Residents have a right to meet with religious leaders, family members, ombudsmen, legal representatives, or any other person.

7. ____ Residents may have a limited number of personal possessions, but they must be approved by facility staff.

8. ____ Person-centered care is related to Residents' Rights because it promotes individual preferences, choices, dignity, and interests.

9. ____ Healthcare workers provide person-centered care by making decisions based on what they would want if they were in the resident's position.

10. ____ Residents can only refuse medications that are not considered critical to their health.

6. Discuss HIPAA, abuse and neglect, and other legal issues

Matching

Match each term with one of the examples below. Use each letter only once.

1. ____ Abuse
2. ____ Diversion
3. ____ Fraud
4. ____ Health Insurance Portability and Accountability Act (HIPAA) requirements
5. ____ Malpractice
6. ____ Mandated reporter
7. ____ Neglect
8. ____ Negligence
9. ____ Protected health information (PHI)

(A) Documenting that a medication was administered when it was not

(B) A person's medical record number

(C) A medication aide who sees a coworker abuse a resident

(D) Administering a medication to the wrong resident because of failure to correctly identify the resident

(E) Stealing a resident's medication and selling it

(F) Not discussing a resident's care with anyone outside the care team

(G) Shaking a resident out of frustration

(H) A provider dismisses a resident's repeated complaints of severe pain and the resident dies from an untreated infection

(I) Residents with incontinence do not have briefs changed promptly or perineal care performed carefully on days when an LTCF is understaffed

Short Answer

10. Mrs. Flores is a new resident at Hartman Hills. MA Angelica has noticed that every time her son visits, Mrs. Flores is agitated before he arrives and very quiet for the rest of the day. When he visits, he closes the door and does not allow anyone to enter. What, if anything, should Angelica do?

____

____

____

11. MA Elianna sees a coworker pulling a resident to move faster on the way to the dining area. She has overheard this same coworker speaking harshly to multiple residents, using rude language and a raised voice. Elianna reports her observations to her supervisor and the supervisor tells her it is not something Elianna should concern herself with. What should Elianna do next? Why?

____

____

Name: ______________________________

____

____

7. Explain laws related to controlled substances

Multiple Choice

1. Controlled substances are defined, or *scheduled* based on
   (A) The route by which they are administered (by mouth, by injection, etc.)
   (B) How often they are seized in law enforcement raids
   (C) Their level of abuse risk and whether or not they have a medical use
   (D) The number of documented cases of abuse or addiction

2. All Schedule I drugs
   (A) Are considered to have the lowest potential for abuse
   (B) Are considered to have the highest potential for abuse
   (C) Can be administered if two providers agree they should be prescribed
   (D) Are illegal drugs given by injection

3. Policies and procedures for handling controlled substances in an LTCF are
   (A) Defined in detail by federal law
   (B) Defined in detail by state law
   (C) Defined by the facility but must follow state law
   (D) Based on the preferences of the facility administrator

4. Which of the following is true?
   (A) All states ban MAs from administering or handling any kind of controlled substance.
   (B) MAs may administer but not count controlled substances.
   (C) MAs may count but not administer controlled substances.
   (D) State rules vary as to whether MAs can administer or count controlled substances.

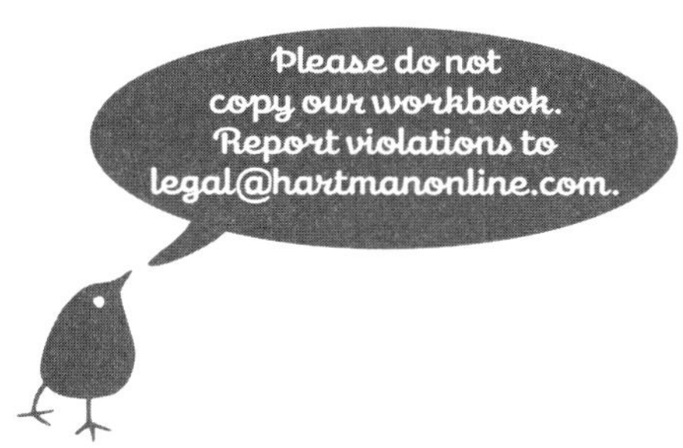

Name: ______________________

3

Medication Basics

1. Define *pharmacology* and related terms

Crossword

Across

2. How a drug moves from where it is administered to the bloodstream
5. How a drug is broken down by the body as time passes
6. The branch of pharmacology that studies what a drug does to the body
7. How a drug moves from the bloodstream to the tissues of the body
8. How a drug exits the body

Down

1. The organ that does most of the work of breaking down a drug in the body
3. The branch of pharmacology that studies what the body does to the drug
4. The branch of medicine that studies the uses and effects of drugs

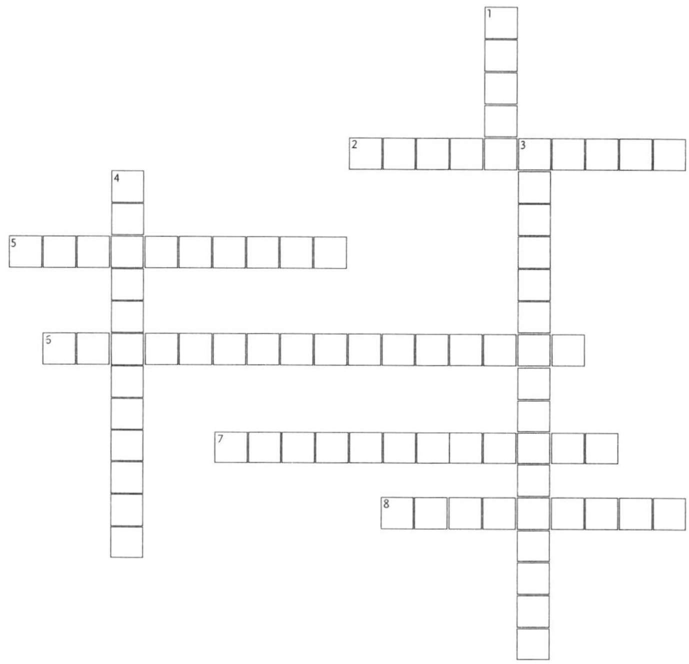

Fill in the Blank

9. One goal of pharmacology is ____________________ new ________________ to help fight diseases.
10. Unwanted ___________________ ___________________ are changes caused by a medication that are unpleasant or harmful.
11. A drug's efficacy is its success in ___________________ ___________________.
12. The effect of a drug on a specific person is called its *clinical effect* or its ___________________ ___________________.

Name: ____________________

2. Identify types of liquid medications

Matching

Use each letter only once.

1. ____ Aerosol
2. ____ Drops
3. ____ Elixir
4. ____ Spray
5. ____ Solution
6. ____ Suspension
7. ____ Syrup
8. ____ Tincture

(A) A liquid pushed through the air in tiny drops

(B) A very small amount of liquid given by dropper

(C) A medication in a solution of sugar or other sweetener and water

(D) A clear, thin flavored liquid, often containing alcohol

(E) A fine spray or mist containing particles suspended in a gas

(F) An extract, usually of a plant material, dissolved in alcohol

(G) A solid, liquid, or gas dissolved in a liquid

(H) A liquid mixture containing drug particles that are not completely dissolved

Short Answer

9. What is one advantage of liquid medications? What is one disadvantage?

____

____

____

____

____

____

10. Which type of liquid medication must be shaken or stirred? Why?

____

____

____

____

3. Identify types of solid and semisolid medications

Multiple Choice

1. This type of tablet is covered by a thin film that protects it from stomach acid:
   (A) Oral disintegrating tablet
   (B) Effervescent tablet
   (C) Buccal tablet
   (D) Enteric-coated tablet

2. This type of medication may be used externally by applying it to the skin or internally by stirring it into a liquid or food.
   (A) Lozenge
   (B) Caplet
   (C) Powder
   (D) Scored tablet

3. Delayed-release tablets should not be
   (A) Crushed or broken/split
   (B) Given by mouth
   (C) Given with beverages other than water
   (D) Given to residents older than 80

4. What is the difference between sublingual, buccal, and oral disintegrating tablets?
   (A) They are different names for the same form of medication.
   (B) They are placed in different parts of the mouth.
   (C) They are digested in different ways.
   (D) They are made for patients of different ages.

5. A medication with an unpleasant taste may be easier to take when it is in this form:
   (A) Oral disintegrating tablet
   (B) Chewable tablet
   (C) Film-coated tablet
   (D) Scored tablet

6. Which of these answer choices includes terms with the same or very similar meanings?
   (A) Film-coated, enteric-coated, effervescent
   (B) Controlled release, extended release, long-acting
   (C) Caplet, troche, capsule
   (D) Chewable, effervescent, disintegrating

True or False

7. _____ Ointment is the thinnest type of semisolid medication.
8. _____ A suppository is a medication form that is inserted into the rectum or vagina.
9. _____ A medicated patch contains a semisolid or liquid form of medication that is absorbed through the skin.
10. _____ Pastes are greasy and provide protective or lubricating effects.
11. _____ Liniments provide moisture and do not contain medication.
12. _____ A topical drug is applied to a body surface.
13. _____ Semisolid medications may be soft and squishy or may have a consistency between solid and liquid.

4. Understand basic medication terminology and abbreviations

Short Answer

1. What is the difference between a prescription drug and an over-the-counter drug?

____

____

____

____

2. How is a drug's brand name selected?

____

____

3. What difference may there be between the brand name and generic forms of the same drug?

____

____

4. When the Medication Safety Board reviews drug packaging and labeling, what risk are they working to decrease?

____

____

5. Why might the use of some abbreviations or symbols increase the risk of medication errors?

____

____

____

____

6. Choose one of the abbreviations listed in Table 3-1 in the textbook (error-prone abbreviations). Describe a situation in which misunderstanding of the abbreviation could cause a medication error.

____

____

____

____

Fill in the Blank

7. Several drugs have names that ______________________ or ______________________ similar. This can cause a problem sometimes called drug name ______________________.
8. Facilities may customize computer screens to prevent ______________________ drug names from appearing one after another in a list.
9. The purpose of a drug is known as the drug's ______________________.

10. It is important for MAs to know where to find a current ______________________ ______________________ book, website, or database, which lists all prescription drugs and their indications.

5. Identify common routes of medication administration

Short Answer

Make a check mark (✓) next to medication forms given by routes in which a drug enters the body and is absorbed through the digestive tract.

1. ____ Intravenous injection
2. ____ Extended-release capsule
3. ____ Syrup
4. ____ Sublingual tablet
5. ____ Subcutaneous injection
6. ____ Suppository
7. ____ Eye ointment
8. ____ Chewable tablet
9. ____ Patch medication
10. ____ Buccal film
11. ____ Effervescent tablet
12. ____ Ear drops

Matching

Letters may be used more than once.

13. ____ The most commonly used medication route
14. ____ May also be called the *optic route*
15. ____ Involves the use of a patch placed on the skin
16. ____ May be intradermal, subcutaneous, intramuscular, or intravenous
17. ____ Absorption usually begins in the mouth and continues in the digestive tract
18. ____ Along with the rectal route, the route that may involve inserting a suppository
19. ____ Involves placing drops in the ear
20. ____ May involve administering drops, gel, or ointment
21. ____ Medication is inserted through the anus
22. ____ Often administered using a handheld device with a mouthpiece
23. ____ Sprayed droplets are absorbed through mucous membranes in the nose
24. ____ Most states do not allow MAs to administer
25. ____ Nebulization route is similar to this route

(A) Inhalation route
(B) Injection routes
(C) Nasal route
(D) Ocular route
(E) Oral route
(F) Otic route
(G) Rectal route
(H) Transdermal route
(I) Topical route
(J) Vaginal route

6. Discuss factors that may affect how the body uses medication

True or False

1. ____ Prescription drugs cause the same effects in every person who takes them.
2. ____ A person's sex assigned at birth can affect the way their body uses medication.
3. ____ Body weight is the only factor a provider considers when setting the dose for a prescription drug.

Name: ______________________________

4. ____ The lungs and the heart are the organs most likely to be affected if a drug accumulates in a person's body.

5. ____ Infants are more sensitive to medications than older children and adults.

6. ____ Some drugs are more or less active based on the amount of body fat a person has.

7. ____ A person's diet does not affect how a drug works in the person's body.

8. ____ A patient who feels confident in a medication's ability to improve health is more likely to experience positive results.

Short Answer

9. Choose two of the "false" statements from exercises 1–8. Rewrite the statements so that they are correct. Give extra information if you can.

____

____

____

____

____

____

____

____

____

____

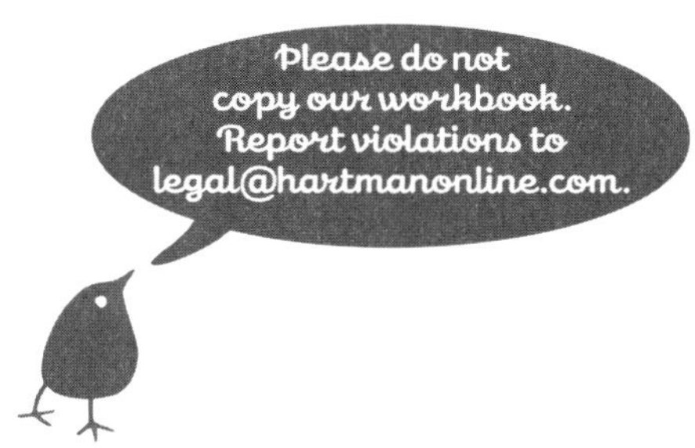

Name: ______________________________

4

Medication Orders and Documentation

1. Describe the different ways medications can be ordered

Multiple Choice

1. Who usually administers medications in a hospital?
   (A) A nurse
   (B) A patient care technician
   (C) A medication aide
   (D) A doctor

2. Which of the following is usually true of a medication order given over the phone?
   (A) It is not valid
   (B) It must be given by an authorized provider to a licensed healthcare professional
   (C) It must be given directly to a pharmacist
   (D) It must be given by an authorized provider but can be received by any person with training in a healthcare field

3. Podiatrists, dentists, and optometrists
   (A) Are some of the providers with the authority to order medications
   (B) Must have a physician (MD) approve any medication they order
   (C) Can order medications for stable, healthy patients with routine illnesses
   (D) Can order medications in a medical emergency

4. MAs cannot receive oral medication orders or administer ______________ medications.
   (A) Routine
   (B) Antiviral
   (C) Chemotherapy
   (D) Stat

2. List the elements of a complete medication order

Fill in the Blank

1. When a controlled medication is ordered, the prescriber's ________________ number must be included.

2. A medication order may use the ________________ or ________________ name of the drug.

3. The amount of active ingredient in one unit of a medication is the ________________ of the drug.

4. Whether a medication is a syrup, a suspension, a tablet, etc., is the ________________ ________________.

5. The ________________ is the amount of medication a patient takes at one time.

6. Directions for use of a medication include whether the medication is to be administered on a regular schedule or ________________.

7. If refills are allowed, a medication order indicates ________________ ________________ and over what period of time.

8. Each time a medication is given to a resident, the MA must confirm
   - right ________________
   - right ________________
   - right ________________
   - right ________________
   - right ________________

   All of this information is provided in the ________________ ________________.

Name: ______________________

3. Explain documentation of medication administration

Short Answer

1. What does *MAR* stand for? What does *eMAR* stand for?

____

____

____

2. For a routine (not PRN) medication, what information must be provided on the MAR?

____

____

____

____

____

____

3. What must be included on the MAR for PRN medications?

____

____

____

4. Why does medication administration need to be documented carefully? List at least two reasons.

____

____

____

____

____

5. How does an MA usually document administration of a drug on a paper MAR?

____

6. How does an eMAR identify a user?

____

____

True or False

7. ____ If a resident refuses a medication, it does not need to be documented in the MAR.

8. ____ In some facilities, follow-up documentation is required after a PRN medication is administered to indicate whether the problem was resolved.

9. ____ Documentation of medication administration should be performed when medications are prepared, before they are taken to the residents.

10. ____ MAs should never document for another person or ask another person to document for them.

11. ____ If a medication is administered but not documented, legally speaking the resident did not receive the medication.

12. ____ A MAR may include information such as the resident's room number and provider's name. An eMAR may include a photo of the resident.

4. Explain the controlled substances medication log

Multiple Choice

1. According to the CDC, what percentage of drug overdose deaths in 2023 were from any form of opioid, legal or illegal?
   (A) 25%
   (B) 50%
   (C) 75%
   (D) 90%

2. What two measures are a common part of screening for new employees at a healthcare facility and may reduce the chances of employees abusing opioids or other drugs?
   (A) Background checks and drug screening
   (B) Lie detector tests and background checks
   (C) Background checks and review of school records
   (D) Drug screening and submission of three character statements

3. In a long-term care facility, controlled medications are generally kept in
   (A) An automated dispensing cabinet that only the charge nurse can access
   (B) A double-locking storage area
   (C) The locked bedside table of the resident to whom they are prescribed
   (D) Rotating (constantly changing) locations determined by the charge nurse

4. How many people must be present when a controlled substance count is performed?
   (A) One
   (B) Two
   (C) Two, and the facility administrator must be one of the two
   (D) Three

5. The amount of a controlled substance before it is dispensed and the amount remaining after it is dispensed are called
   (A) The starting balance and the ending balance
   (B) The initial balance and the final balance
   (C) The first balance and the last balance
   (D) The countback balance and the forward balance

6. Which of the following is a feature of some eMAR systems that can help with management of controlled medications?
   (A) They keep an ongoing count of controlled medications.
   (B) They do not allow MAs to access records for residents who have controlled medications prescribed.
   (C) They suggest alternative medications that do not carry a risk of abuse or addiction.
   (D) They automatically dial the number of the resident's provider to confirm that each administration of the medication is necessary.

5. Describe how to observe and report accurately

Short Answer

1. What type of information is most helpful to the nurse and the care team?

____

2. What is the difference between objective and subjective information?

____

____

____

____

3. Why are vital signs important?

____

____

____

Name: ______________________________

4. Why might an MA be required to measure vital signs before a medication is administered?

____

____

____

____

____

5. List five observations about a resident that an MA must report to the nurse immediately.

____

____

____

____

____

____

____

6. What happens during an anaphylactic reaction?

____

____

____

____

True or False

7. ____ Hypertensive crisis occurs when systolic blood pressure is higher than 180 mm Hg or diastolic blood pressure is over 120 mm Hg.

8. ____ If a resident's blood pressure is above normal, an MA can choose not to administer medications until a normal reading is taken.

9. ____ An MA's observations about residents can help the nurse assess how the resident is responding to a medication.

10. ____ A visible rash is an example of subjective information and a resident's report of itching is an example of objective information.

6. Discuss how to resolve questions about medication orders

Complete the Sentence

In each of the following sentences, underline the correct choice between the words or phrases in italics.

1. If a resident's MAR is missing required information, the MA should contact *their supervisor | the resident's provider.*

2. If the MAR is missing information, the MA *should administer the medication only if it is one the resident has taken before | should not administer the medication.*

3. If an MA finds it strange that a particular medication is ordered for a resident, they should *understand that it is beyond their scope of practice to ask questions | confirm the order with the nurse before administering the drug.*

4. One reliable source for information about medications is *a facility-approved website | a more experienced MA.*

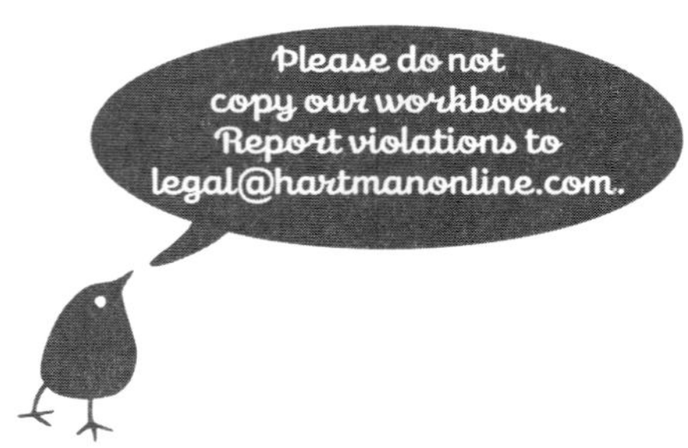

5

Medication Dosage

1. Discuss medication dose conversion

Multiple Choice

1. How should liquid cough medication be measured in a healthcare setting?
   (A) By teaspoon
   (B) By drop
   (C) By liter
   (D) By milliliter

2. Which of these tasks is beyond an MA's scope of practice?
   (A) Checking a resident's MAR before administering a medication
   (B) Reporting to a nurse if a medication dose seems very high or very low
   (C) Calculating how many milliliters of a liquid medication to give a resident when the MAR gives the number of milligrams of active ingredient that should be administered
   (D) Measuring the ordered amount of a liquid medication before administering it to a resident

3. When a healthcare professional converts a medication dose
   (A) The prescribed amount must not change
   (B) The prescribed amount goes down
   (C) The prescribed amount goes up
   (D) The prescribed amount changes based on which units of measurement are involved

2. Explain the most common measurement systems for medication dosing

Short Answer

For each item below, write A for apothecaries' system, M for metric system, and H for household measurements.

1. ____ The standard measurement system in health care
2. ____ One of the oldest forms of measurement
3. ____ Teaspoons and tablespoons are units in this system
4. ____ May be more familiar to residents than other systems
5. ____ Based on multiples of 10
6. ____ Scruples and drams are units in this system
7. ____ Allows for the most accurate calculations
8. ____ Weight is measured in pounds and ounces
9. ____ Uses Roman numerals
10. ____ Basic unit for volume is the liter

Fill in the Blank

11. __________ milligrams (mg) = 1 gram (g)
12. 1000 g = __________ kilogram(s) (kg)
13. 1000 microliters = __________ milliliter (mL)
14. __________ mL = 1 liter (L)

15. 0.5 g = __________ mg

16. 0.022 L = __________ mL

17. 2 teaspoons = __________ mL

18. One reason household spoons should never be used for administering medications is that they _______________ _______________ _______________.

3. Explain dosage range

Matching

Use each letter only once.

1. _____ Clinical trials
2. _____ Dosage range
3. _____ Narrow therapeutic index drug
4. _____ Therapeutic dose
5. _____ Toxicity

(A) A medication dose that has the desired effect on the patient

(B) The upper limit is the maximum amount of a drug that can be administered without toxic effects; the lower limit is the minimum amount of a drug that has the desired effect on the patient

(C) Part of the drug development process in which a drug is given to patients who are monitored carefully to observe the effects

(D) A poisoning effect

(E) A medication for which the gap between the highest safe dose and the lowest effective dose is very small

Fill in the Blank

6. ______________________ and medications that control ______________________ are examples of narrow therapeutic index drugs.

7. ______________________, diabetes, heart failure, and ______________________ ______________________ are among the most common conditions seen in long-term care facilities.

8. Because MAs have frequent one-on-one contact with residents, they are in a good position to ______________________ and ______________________ changes.

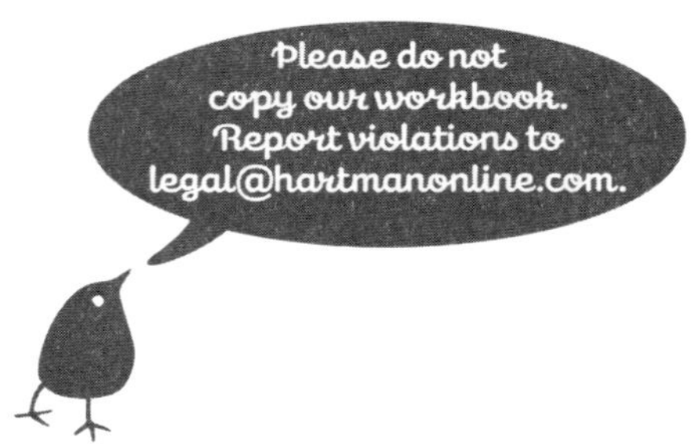

6

Medication Side Effects, Reactions, and Interactions

1. Discuss medication side effects

Multiple Choice

1. As a medication moves through the body, what do *receptors* do?
   (A) They surround and remove drug particles from the body.
   (B) They receive chemical information from the drug and may be activated or inactivated.
   (C) They increase thirst, which helps a person drink more water and process the drug.
   (D) They carry the drug to the part of the body that benefits from its effect.

2. Drug effects that occur when the medication affects receptors that are not the treatment target tissues are called
   (A) Therapeutic effects
   (B) Complicating effects
   (C) Diversion effects
   (D) Side effects

3. Side effects are possible
   (A) At any dose
   (B) Only when the dose administered is toward the top of the safe dosage range
   (C) Only when a dose is increased
   (D) Only when a dose is decreased

4. Side effects are mostly predictable because
   (A) They are planned by the drug developer
   (B) They are extreme versions of the intended effects of the drug
   (C) They are studied during clinical trials
   (D) A facility keeps a list of side effects residents experience with each drug

5. Most side effects
   (A) Do not require any action
   (B) Are dangerous to residents
   (C) Are serious enough to prevent people from taking a drug
   (D) Are psychosomatic, or caused by a person's thoughts about the drug

6. The nurse administered COVID-19 vaccinations to residents in the morning. In the afternoon, many of the residents told MA Sarai they needed her to ask the nurse to approve Tylenol for sore arms. This is an example of
   (A) A systemic side effect of the vaccine
   (B) A local side effect of the vaccine
   (C) An anaphylactic reaction to the vaccine
   (D) The therapeutic effect of the vaccine

7. This class of drug can have local side effects when it is given by inhalation and systemic side effects, sometimes severe, when taken orally for an extended time:
   (A) Anticoagulants
   (B) Corticosteroids
   (C) Oral contraceptives
   (D) Antidepressants

8. Which of the following is true?
   (A) Side effects are always unwanted.
   (B) Side effects are the same for every person who takes a medication.
   (C) Side effects of a medication for one condition may be used to treat a different condition.
   (D) Side effects always stop happening as a person's body gets used to a medication.

2. Discuss adverse reactions to medications

True or False

1. ____ *Adverse reaction* is another term for *side effect.*
2. ____ One predictable adverse reaction is excessive bleeding caused by an anticoagulant drug.
3. ____ *Idiosyncratic* is another word for *expected.*
4. ____ An allergic reaction to a drug is a type of side effect.
5. ____ Antibiotics are a type of drug that may cause allergic reactions.
6. ____ Allergic reactions to drugs are always severe.
7. ____ If a resident is going to have an anaphylactic reaction to a medication, it always happens within 15 minutes of taking the drug for the first time.
8. ____ EpiPen is a brand name for a medication that may be administered when a resident is having an anaphylactic reaction.
9. ____ A paradoxical reaction happens when a drug causes an effect that is opposite of what is expected.
10. ____ Because adverse reactions are predictable, MAs can know when to watch for them.

Short Answer

11. Why are adverse reactions a good illustration of why an MA must always be alert and observant while administering medications?

____

____

____

____

____

12. What is the first thing an MA should do if a resident shows signs of anaphylaxis?

____

13. MA Sarai has noticed that a resident who has a PRN order for a medication to calm anxiety becomes more agitated after taking the medication. What should Sarai do? If the resident's agitation is caused by the medication, what type of adverse reaction is this?

____

____

____

____

3. Explain drug tolerance

Fill in the Blank

1. Drug tolerance occurs when a patient no longer has the same ____________ from the same ____________ of a medication.
2. Drug tolerance is different from drug ____________ or ____________.
3. Tolerance may develop when receptors targeted by the drug ____________ ____________ the desired response. It may also happen when the drug begins clearing from the body ____________ ____________.
4. Residents who take a number of medications regularly may be ____________ likely to develop drug tolerance.
5. Cross tolerance happens when a person has developed tolerance to one drug and also shows tolerance to other drugs in the ____________ drug ____________.
6. There are both ____________ and ____________ aspects to drug addiction.

7. A person with a drug dependence may have ______________________symptoms such as headache, nausea, and vomiting when the drug is not in the person's system.

Short Answer

8. List three drug classes to which a resident may be especially likely to develop tolerance.

____

____

____

9. Who decides how best to manage the situation when a resident develops a drug tolerance?

____

10. How might an MA's observing and reporting help identify drug tolerance in a resident?

____

____

____

____

4. Describe drug interactions

Matching

Use each letter only once.

1. ____ Addition
2. ____ Antagonism
3. ____ Drug-disease interaction
4. ____ Drug-drug interaction
5. ____ Drug-nutrient interaction
6. ____ Interaction
7. ____ Potentiation
8. ____ Synergism

(A) In pharmacology, a situation in which a substance or condition changes the way a drug works in a person's body

(B) A situation in which one drug changes the effects of another

(C) A drug interaction in which the action of one drug decreases or cancels the effects of the other drug

(D) A drug interaction in which the action of one drug increases the effects of the other drug or makes its effects last longer

(E) A situation in which a health condition affects how a drug works in a person's body

(F) A drug interaction in which the combined effect of two or more drugs is greater than the sum of the effects of each drug alone

(G) A drug interaction in which the combined effects of two drugs equal the sum of the effects of each drug alone

(H) A situation in which a food, beverage, or dietary supplement changes the effect of a drug

Scenarios

Read each scenario below and then write the name of the type of drug interaction involved.

9. Mrs. Adamski has hypertension and takes medication to lower her blood pressure. When MA Sammie takes Mrs. Adamski's blood pressure during a lunchtime medication pass, she finds that it is very low. She sees two empty cans of grapefruit juice on Mrs. Adamski's bedside table and asks her about them. Mrs. Adamski tells Sammie that her son stopped by on his way to work and gave her the grapefruit juice. She meant to save a can for the next day, but she drank both because she loves it so much.

   What type of interaction may be happening?

____

10. Mr. Cano takes a diuretic medication to lower his blood pressure and reduce swelling in his legs and feet. He took ibuprofen for a muscle strain and found that his feet were more swollen than usual and his blood pressure was a bit higher.

   What type of interaction may be happening?

____

Name: ____________________

11. Mrs. Morgan loves greens and eats greens every day. During the holidays she had many visitors who brought her special foods, and she did not eat her greens as often. Mrs. Morgan takes the anticoagulant warfarin and has her blood tested regularly to be sure her blood clotting times stay in the right range. When she was tested right after the holidays her results were out of range.

    What type of interaction may be happening?

____

12. Mr. Mustain has mild asthma and stage 2 hypertension. When he begins a new type of medication to control his blood pressure, his asthma gets worse.

    What type of interaction may be happening?

____

True or False

13. ____ Herbal supplements never interact with prescription medications because they are natural.

14. ____ Alcohol should be avoided when taking medications that stimulate or depress the nervous system.

15. ____ Vitamin C is the nutrient in leafy green vegetables that may change the effects of the anticoagulant warfarin.

16. ____ Calcium-containing foods may reduce the effectiveness of some antibiotics.

17. ____ MAs should not advise residents about possible drug interactions.

18. ____ Drug interactions can be especially serious when narrow therapeutic index drugs are involved.

7

Medication Safety

1. Explain the "rights" of medication administration

Short Answer

After each item below, list the related "right" of medication administration: right resident, right medication, right dose, right route, right time, or right documentation. Each right may be used more than once.

1. Mr. Murray's medication must be taken on an empty stomach, so when she takes morning medications to residents, MA Naomi always makes sure he gets his medication before breakfast.

____

2. Mrs. Reddy has a headache. The nurse has assessed her pain and assigned MA Frances to administer acetaminophen. Mrs. Reddy's MAR lists 650 mg of acetaminophen every 4 hours as needed for headache. Frances sees that the facility's stock medications include 325-mg and 500-mg tablets and prepares two 325-mg tablets for Mrs. Reddy.

____

3. Every time MA Corey brings medications to residents, she says, "Pretend I have amnesia and tell me your first and last names so I can make sure I give you the right medicine."

____

4. MA Jess knows that eye drops and ear drops may look similar, so every time she is administering these types of medications she checks carefully to be sure she is using the correct bottle.

____

5. MA Jasmine carries a tablet computer with her during medication administration and always marks each resident's eMAR after they take their medications and before she leaves the room.

____

6. There are two residents at Hartman Hills with very similar names: Carolina Garcia and Caroline Garcia. When MA Elena is preparing and administering medications she double-checks the names and dates of birth for these residents especially carefully.

____

7. Hartman Hills' eMAR system uses capital letters to emphasize differences in similar drug names. This helps MAs avoid confusing one medication for another.

____

8. Mr. Law has the flu and is running a fever. He tells MA Matt that he could really use some Advil (ibuprofen) for his aches and fever. Matt knows that Mr. Law takes an anticoagulant and that ibuprofen could increase his bleeding risk. Matt sees that acetaminophen is listed on Mr. Law's MAR as a PRN medication and asks the nurse if she could assess Mr. Law so he can receive the medication.

____

9. Mrs. Shriver had been taking oral anti-nausea medications due to cancer treatment, but she was unable to swallow them because her nausea was severe. Her provider ordered the same medication, but in the form of a patch. Now instead of administering pills 3 times each day, MA Donna places a patch on Mrs.

Shriver's arm and does not change it for 3 days.

____

10. Mrs. Stephens' provider is gradually lowering the dose of a blood pressure medication she takes. She used to take 10-mg tablets and now she takes 5-mg tablets. MA Madison checks the medication carefully before administering it.

____

2. Identify information needed about the resident and the medication prior to administration

Complete the Sentence

1. Before administering some medications, an MA may be required to *check certain vital signs | perform a urine dipstick test.*
2. A resident's warfarin dose may be adjusted by the provider based on the *resident's blood pressure measurement | results of a blood test.*
3. Before administering a drug, the MA should be aware of a resident's *DNR status | known allergies.*
4. Not checking blood pressure before administering a medication that is supposed to be held if the resident's blood pressure is normal or low can cause *an increased risk of falls | anaphylaxis.*
5. MAs can only administer established medications to *stable residents | critically ill residents.*
6. The most common resident identifiers checked before medication is administered are *full name and room number | full name and date of birth.*

Matching

For each of the following types of information about a drug, write the letter of the example that is the best match. (Note that the examples do not all refer to the same drug.) Use each letter only once.

7. _____ Adverse effects
8. _____ Effect
9. _____ Indication
10. _____ Interactions
11. _____ Length of time to take effect
12. _____ Name
13. _____ Side effects
14. _____ Special instructions

(A) Lasix (furosemide)

(B) Increases levels of certain chemicals in the blood by blocking their absorption

(C) May cause nausea or diarrhea

(D) Used to treat diabetes

(E) Should not be taken with grapefruit or grapefruit juice

(F) Should be taken with food

(G) Anaphylaxis caused by an antibiotic

(H) 45 minutes to 1 hour

3. Explain medication contraindications

True or False

1. _____ A *contraindication* relates to the type of medication best suited to treat a resident's condition.
2. _____ An MA may hold a medication if they believe it is contraindicated for a resident.
3. _____ MAs should know contraindications for drugs they administer.
4. _____ Contraindications are always listed in a resident's MAR.
5. _____ A medication that helps to maintain normal blood sugar levels would most likely be contraindicated for a resident with diabetes.

4. Discuss safe medication storage

Multiple Choice

1. Which of the following is a type of facility where medications are more likely to be stored in each resident's unit?
   (A) A traditional long-term care facility/nursing home
   (B) A rehabilitation center
   (C) An assisted living facility
   (D) A hospital

2. Medications should be stored in a ____________________ area away from ____________________.
   (A) Humid, children
   (B) Dry, sunlight
   (C) Warm, drafts
   (D) Cold, liquids

3. This is another term for distributing medications to residents:
   (A) Passing medications
   (B) Pressing medications
   (C) Setting up medications
   (D) Assigning medications

4. Medications that are not stored properly
   (A) Can lose their effectiveness or even become toxic
   (B) May change color or look different but still have the same effect
   (C) Must be discarded or destroyed by the ordering provider
   (D) Should be used up as quickly as possible

5. Medication storage rooms or carts must have separate storage for
   (A) Tablets and capsules
   (B) Syrups and suspensions
   (C) Liquid and solid oral medications
   (D) Topical and oral medications

6. Over-the-counter medications kept on hand for PRN use may be called
   (A) Occasional medications
   (B) Reserved medications
   (C) Routine medications
   (D) Stock medications

7. During an MA's shift, keys to medication rooms or carts
   (A) Should be left in the lock if the MA will need to access the medications repeatedly
   (B) Should be left on the counter of the nurses' station where the MA can easily reach them
   (C) Should be kept under the MA's direct control at all times
   (D) Should be placed on the bedside table of the resident whose medications will be administered last so the MA does not forget to lock everything after they are done

8. In addition to handwashing, an MA may use a sink in the medication storage room to
   (A) Dilute medications to the ordered strength
   (B) Wash supplies and equipment after using them
   (C) Dispose of medications that residents have refused
   (D) Dissolve tablets or other solid medications in water when a resident cannot swallow pills

9. When medications are stored in a refrigerator they must be
   (A) Kept in the crisper drawer to maintain freshness
   (B) Removed from their packaging first to prevent moisture buildup
   (C) Kept in a separate refrigerator from food
   (D) Kept in sealed, insulated containers

10. What should an MA do if the temperature of the medication storage area does not seem to be correct?
   (A) Report to a supervisor
   (B) Place a maintenance order for repair of the heating or cooling system
   (C) Request a fan (if it is too hot) or space heater (if it is too cold)
   (D) Move the medications into each resident's room

Name: ______________________________

5. Describe safe medication disposal

Fill in the Blank

Fill in the blank to complete this list of situations in which a medication must be discarded or destroyed.

1. A resident ________________ the facility and will not ________________.
2. A resident's treatment plan has ________________.
3. A medication that was prepared must be ________________ due to resident's condition.
4. A resident develops a(n) ________________ or other adverse reaction from a medication.
5. The medication is past its ________________ ________________.
6. A resident ________________ the medication after it is prepared.
7. The medication has been ________________ or damaged.
8. A resident ________________.

True or False

9. ____ If a medication is disposed of or destroyed for reasons that do not involve a resident (e.g., it fell on the floor), the disposal does not need to be documented or reported.
10. ____ Proper disposal of medications also involves protecting resident privacy.
11. ____ MAs are not allowed to dispose of medications for any reason in any state, but should understand the processes involved.
12. ____ When controlled medications are disposed of/destroyed, two staff members are usually required to be present.

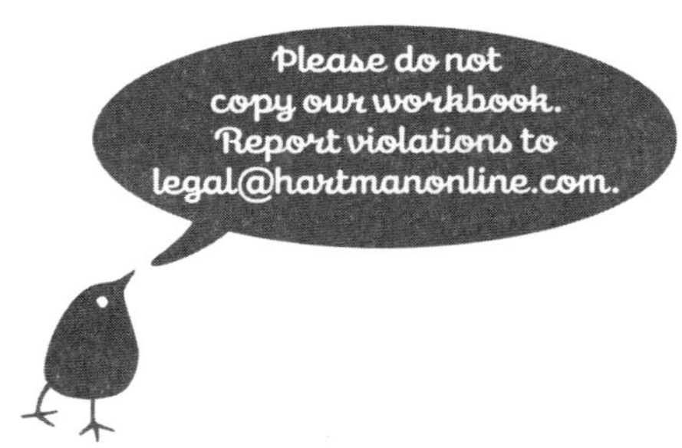

8

Preparation and Administration of Medication

1. Describe systems for packaging and distributing medications

Multiple Choice

1. In a long-term care facility, which of these types of medication is most likely to be in unit dose packaging?
   (A) Emergency supplies of commonly used prescription medications
   (B) A medication that a resident has taken daily for years and will continue to take
   (C) Nonprescription topical medications
   (D) Nonprescription oral medications in liquid form

2. What is the difference between unit dose packaging and a blister pack/punch card?
   (A) Unit dose packaging is for liquid medications and blister packs/punch cards are for tablets and capsules.
   (B) Unit dose packaging is for over-the-counter medications and blister packs/punch cards are for prescription medications.
   (C) Unit dose packaging contains a single dose of a drug and blister packs/punch cards have multiple doses of the same drug on a single card.
   (D) Unit dose packaging contains only one type of medication and blister packs/punch cards always contain every type of medication a resident takes on a single card.

3. Which of the following is a common system of medication administration at LTCFs?
   (A) Residents line up at the door of the medication storage room at set times each day and MAs prepare and administer medications for each one in turn.
   (B) MAs accompany a provider on rounds each day and the provider sends the MA to prepare medications for each resident after a consultation.
   (C) MAs wait in a medication storage area and nurses and other staff send residents to receive their medications at the correct times.
   (D) MAs take a medication storage cart from room to room and administer medications at set times each day.

4. If a facility has any medications in traditional packaging, they are most likely to be
   (A) Powerful antibiotics
   (B) Common over-the-counter medications
   (C) Drugs that control diabetes
   (D) Controlled medications

5. This is one feature that unit dose packages and blister packs/punch cards usually have in common:
   (A) Foil backing
   (B) The ability to reuse packages
   (C) They are created for a specific resident
   (D) They are for emergency use

2. Discuss how to prevent infection while administering medications

Fill in the Blank

1. *Aseptic* means ________________ ________________ pathogens.
2. Before preparing or administering medications, the MA should ________________ ________________ thoroughly.
3. Hand hygiene should be performed after administering a ________________ medication.
4. Surfaces on which medications are prepared should be cleaned regularly with facility-approved ________________.
5. If a medication tray is set down outside a medication room, it must be ________________ before it is returned.
6. Souffle cups should be stored with the opening ________________ and handled by the ________________.
7. A paper souffle cup should be used only ________________ ________________ and then ________________.
8. If a medication falls on the floor it must be reported, documented, and ________________. A ________________ ________________ must be prepared.

Short Answer

9. List three medication routes that require an MA to wear gloves during administration.

10. Give at least two examples of other situations when an MA may wear gloves while administering medications.

11. What should MAs check before using a pill splitter or crusher (in addition to making sure the MAR indicates splitting/crushing)?

3. Discuss special considerations when administering medications

Scenarios

Read each scenario below and then write how the MA should respond.

1. Mr. Eubanks has been taking an antibiotic for 3 days. He is supposed to take it for 7 more days. After MA Daria steps in his room, Mr. Eubanks says, "Don't even come in here. That pill is making me sicker than I was before."

2. Mrs. Jabeur prefers for healthcare workers to touch her as little as possible, and she prefers to have female healthcare workers care for her if the care requires touch. MA Alexander is on duty during a time of day when Mrs. Jabeur needs to have a topical medication applied to her lower back.

3. When MA Catherine arrives in Mr. Shelton's room to give him his medications, he asks her why he's still getting a blood pressure pill when his blood pressure has been normal for weeks.

____

____

____

____

____

Short Answer

Make a check mark (✓) next to each correct guideline for administering medications to elderly residents.

4. _____ Encourage residents to take as many medications together as they are able to take. This helps the resident to get the benefit of the medications more quickly and helps the MA stay on schedule.

5. _____ Suggest placing tablets or capsules toward the back of the tongue for easier swallowing.

6. _____ Do not rush residents.

7. _____ Administer medications to residents in the position in which the resident feels most comfortable.

8. _____ If a resident is not on fluid restrictions, encourage the resident to drink more liquid after all drugs have been administered.

9. _____ Leave medications on a resident's bedside table if a resident is sleeping during a medication pass.

10. _____ For residents with swallowing problems, crush all tablets and/or open all capsules and mix the drug with applesauce.

11. _____ Suggest that the resident first sip some liquid to moisten their mouth so that swallowing the medications will be easier.

12. _____ If a resident takes medications with liquid, provide a full cup to allow easy and thorough swallowing.

13. _____ Do not allow residents to do anything for themselves to reduce the chance of errors.

14. _____ Politely check that the resident has swallowed all medications.

4. List steps to follow and safety checks to perform when setting up medications

Multiple Choice

1. During medication setup, when are the first, second, and third safety checks performed?
   (A) When the medication is prescribed, when it is dispensed, and when it is administered
   (B) When the medication is removed from storage, when the dose is removed from its package, and just before it is administered
   (C) When the medication is delivered to the facility, when it is placed in the medication storage area, and just before it is administered
   (D) When the medication is removed from storage, just before it is administered, and before it is documented

2. When medication safety checks are performed, what should the MA keep in mind?
   (A) The "rights" of medication administration
   (B) The need to work quickly
   (C) The indications and possible adverse effects of each drug
   (D) The number of residents still waiting for their medications

3. Which of the following pieces of information is commonly on a prescription label for a liquid medication?
   (A) The number of teaspoons in the ordered dose
   (B) The color of the liquid
   (C) A full list of possible adverse effects
   (D) Instructions for taking the medication

4. When setting up medications the MA should compare information on the medication label to information
   (A) On the resident's MAR
   (B) On the facility's drug reference software
   (C) In the original provider medication order
   (D) On the resident's ADL sheet

5. When setting up medications, the first step to avoiding medication errors is
   (A) Confirming that each resident is ready to receive their medications
   (B) Asking the nurse to double-check the list of residents who will receive medications
   (C) Removing distractions
   (D) Making sure there is a provider in the facility who can check the MA's work

6. What is the first point at which an MA must wash hands during the medication administration process?
   (A) Before beginning setup
   (B) After getting out souffle cups, pill splitters, and any other needed equipment and supplies
   (C) Before entering the first resident's room
   (D) After the first contact with a resident

7. Which of these correctly lists the six "rights" of medication administration as described in the textbook?
   (A) Right time, right indication, right effects, right dose, right route, right ordering provider
   (B) Right manufacturer, right name, right form, right strength, right instructions, right resident
   (C) Right resident, right indication, right safety checks, right dose, right route, right documentation
   (D) Right resident, right medication, right dose, right route, right time, right documentation

True or False

8. ____ A medication cup with markings in tablespoons is the most accurate device for administering liquid medications.

9. ____ If there is any difference between the information on a resident's MAR and the label for a medication being administered to the resident, the MA must tell a supervisor.

10. ____ Using the incorrect strength of a medication can result in a resident getting too much or too little of the drug's active ingredient.

11. ____ When dispensing tablets or capsules from a bottle, the correct technique is for the MA to use one gloved finger to reach in and pull the correct number of pills out.

12. ____ If medications are administered from a medication cart, the final of the three medication safety checks may happen at the patient's bedside.

13. ____ The proper way to pour liquid medications from a bottle is to position the bottle with the label facing upward, toward the palm of the MA's hand.

14. ____ Before administering a medication for the first time, an MA should know the name(s) of the drug, its indications, possible side effects or adverse effects, and common dosage information.

15. ____ Not shaking a liquid medication may affect its texture or taste, but will not affect the dosage.

16. ____ A medication that is past its expiration date should not be administered.

Scenarios

Read the scenarios below and then answer the questions that follow.

MA Harrison is setting up medications and finds that when the label on a new blister pack printed, part of the information was cut off. He can see all of the information clearly except for the strength. The strength of medication listed in the MAR is 250 mg. The label cuts off so that it seems to read *25*, but it is clear that information is missing.

17. What should Harrison do?

____

____

18. Is the answer any different if this is a medication that Harrison has administered to the same resident for a long time and it looks the same as it always has?

____

____

19. Is the answer any different if the resident looks at the medication and confirms that it is correct?

____

____

MA Naomi is doing the third and final safety check on Mr. Cruz's morning medications. She always likes to count the pills in a souffle cup before handing the cup to a resident. When she does this, she notices that there is one less pill in the cup than there should be. She checks all of the punch cards for Mr. Cruz's medications and finds that one pill did not fall out of the packet when she pressed the dose through the foil. She presses that pill into the cup and counts again, finding that she has the correct number of pills.

20. Is it a good idea to count pills in a souffle cup before administering medications? Why or why not?

____

____

____

____

21. Can you think of any other techniques for improving medication safety during setup?

____

____

____

MA Shavon is mixing a powdered medication for a resident. She cannot find the measuring cup she usually uses to measure the liquid that is mixed with the powder. She knows about how far up the glass the mixture usually goes.

22. Is it OK for Shavon to guess at the volume of liquid to use to mix this medication? Why or why not?

____

____

____

____

5. Discuss procedures for medication administration by route

Short Answer

Make a check mark (✓) next to steps an MA always needs to follow before administering any medication.

1. ____ Call the provider to confirm the order
2. ____ Identify the resident correctly, usually by asking the resident to confirm their room number and the name of their provider
3. ____ Position the resident correctly based on the route of administration
4. ____ Don a mask before entering the patient's room
5. ____ Identify the resident correctly, usually by asking the resident to state their full name and date of birth
6. ____ Measure vital signs and/or weight as directed in the MAR
7. ____ Provide a light snack so that the medications do not upset the resident's stomach
8. ____ Introduce themselves and describe what they are going to do

Name: ______________________________

Complete the Sentence

9. Most residents *are not able* | *are able* to place pills in their mouths and swallow them without help.

10. When a resident cannot place pills in her own mouth, the MA should use *a spoon* | *their gloved fingers* to place the pills in the resident's mouth for her.

11. Never leave the room until the resident has *picked up the souffle cup holding his medications* | *swallowed all ordered medications.*

12. Encourage residents to *drink plenty of fluids* | *eat plenty of food* when taking oral medications.

13. Report any doubts or questions a resident has about a medication to *the nurse* | *the resident's provider.*

14. *Reject* | *Respect* a resident's refusal to take a medication.

Multiple Choice

15. In which of the following situations should an MA report to a supervisor and not administer an ordered medication?
    (A) A required vital sign measurement is out of range
    (B) A resident is sleeping when the MA enters the room
    (C) A resident has a visitor when the MA enters the room
    (D) The MA is running short on time to complete the medication pass

16. How should a resident be positioned to swallow oral medications?
    (A) The resident should be mostly upright, elevated to at least 60 degrees
    (B) The resident should be completely upright, elevated to 90 degrees
    (C) The resident should be leaning slightly forward
    (D) The resident should be supine

17. If a resident is taking both solid and liquid medications, which should be administered first?
    (A) The solid medication is administered first
    (B) The liquid medication is administered first
    (C) The medication administered first is whichever one is more convenient for the MA
    (D) The medication administered first is whichever one the resident prefers to take first

18. When should an MA explain the medication administration procedure to a resident?
    (A) Every time a medication is administered
    (B) Only before administering a medication the MA hasn't administered to a particular resident before
    (C) Only before administering a medication to a resident the MA has not met
    (D) Only before administering a medication with possible serious side effects or adverse effects

Short Answer

19. Why should buccal and sublingual medications not be chewed and swallowed?

____

____

____

____

20. When can an MA offer fluids or food after administering a buccal or sublingual medication?

____

____

21. Where is a buccal medication placed to dissolve?

____

____

22. Where is a sublingual medication placed to dissolve?

____

____

True or False

23. _____ All inhaled medications are administered by metered dose inhaler.

24. _____ Oxygen is considered a drug and is usually administered by a nurse.

25. _____ Metered dose inhalers have counters that show the number of inhalations ("puffs") remaining in the canister.

26. _____ If a metered dose inhaler is not primed before it is used for the first time, the resident may not get the correct dose of medication.

27. _____ Even if residents have administered their own inhaled medications for many years, MAs must hold and activate metered dose inhalers for residents who use them.

28. _____ Spacers are only used for pediatric patients.

29. _____ Spacers must be cleaned regularly.

30. _____ Rinsing the mouth with water after inhaled corticosteroids are administered can help prevent a type of fungal infection that is a common side effect associated with these drugs.

31. _____ Nebulizers are all very similar and medications can be administered by nebulizer in all states.

32. _____ When administering a medication by metered dose inhaler, the MA should grip the inhaler in a fist.

33. _____ When a resident is using a spacer with a metered dose inhaler, they should breathe in slowly after the medication is released into the chamber.

34. _____ Timing of inhalation is not as important when administering a medication from an inhaler without a spacer as it is when a spacer is used.

35. _____ Instructions for using a metered dose inhaler often include telling the resident to hold their breath for a short time after inhaling the medication.

36. _____ A metered dose inhaler must be shaken before the medication is administered.

Complete the Sentence

37. Nasal medications are often prescribed to control *allergies and congestion* | *nausea and vomiting.*

38. Nasal drops are best administered with a resident *in prone position* | *in supine position* with their head tilted back.

39. For administration of nasal sprays, the resident should be *lying on his back* | *seated* with his head tilted slightly forward.

40. Nasal *sprays* | *drops* often must be primed before first use, according to manufacturer instructions.

41. When administering nasal drops, the MA should *touch* | *not touch* the dropper to the resident's nostril.

42. MAs should direct nasal drops toward *the outer edge of the nostril* | *the nasal septum.*

Multiple Choice

43. What must an MA always wear while administering ophthalmic medications?
    (A) Gloves
    (B) A mask
    (C) A face shield
    (D) A complete set of PPE

44. What are the two forms of optic medications an MA can administer?
    (A) Sprays and drops
    (B) Drops and injections
    (C) Ointments and drops
    (D) Ointments and sprays

Name: ______________________________

45. Why should an MA wait 5 minutes between administering drops of optic medications if multiple drops are ordered?
    (A) Because the medications sting and it takes time for the resident to recover
    (B) Because the medications are thick and it takes time for a second drop to form in the dropper
    (C) Because the medications take time to absorb and the first drop needs time to absorb before the second is administered
    (D) Because the nurse has to assess whether the first drop was administered correctly before the second drop is administered

46. Eye ointment is administered
    (A) In a circular dab near the inner canthus
    (B) In a line between the eye and the lower eyelid
    (C) In a line between the eye and the upper eyelid
    (D) In a circular dab near the outer canthus

47. When should an MA use a gloved finger to press gently on the inner canthus of a resident's eye?
    (A) Immediately before eye ointment is administered
    (B) Immediately after eye ointment is administered
    (C) Immediately before eye drops are administered
    (D) Immediately after eye drops are administered

48. When administering eye drops, the MA should not
    (A) Tell the resident when the drop will fall
    (B) Wear any form of PPE
    (C) First wash hands with soap and water
    (D) Touch the dropper to the eye

Crossword

Across

49. Before administering ear drops, the MA should use a cotton ball to wipe debris or ______________ from the outer ear

50. Instilling drops so that they run down the side of the ear canal avoids trapping this in the ear canal

51. Do not insert anything in the ear, including cotton ______________

52. Pulling the ear up and back before instilling drops straightens this

Down

53. Wait at least this many minutes after instilling one ear drop before you instill a second drop if one is ordered

54. This may be placed on, but not inserted in, the ear after ear drops are administered

55. A resident may experience this if cold ear drops are instilled in their ear

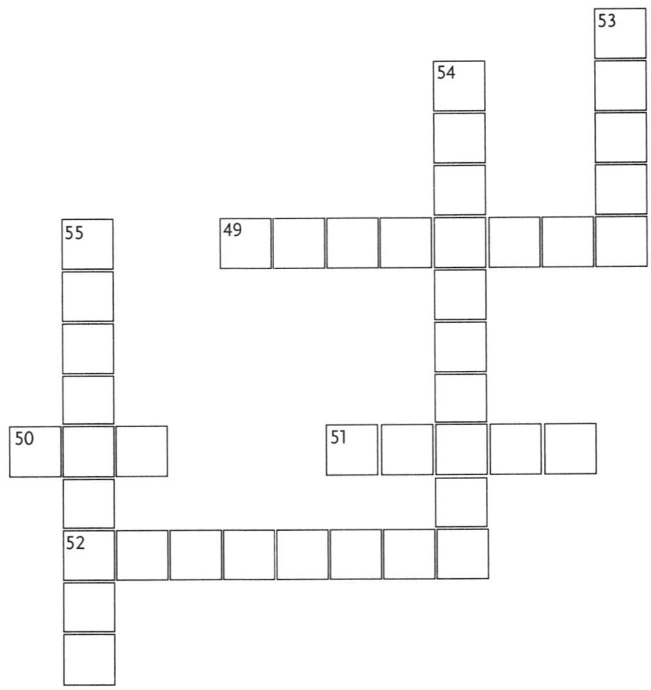

Short Answer

56. What types of topical medication are often rubbed in?

____

57. What type of topical medication is often left on top of the skin as a protecting layer?

____

58. List two applicators that may be used to administer topical medications.

____

____

59. How should the MA protect the resident's privacy when exposing the area where a topical medication will be administered?

___

___

___

60. Why should an MA be careful with the resident's and their own clothing when administering topical medications?

___

___

61. What signs/symptoms may be treated with a medicated soak?

___

___

62. What is the maximum water temperature that should be used for a medicated soak? How should the temperature be tested?

___

___

___

___

True or False

63. ____ Transdermal patch medications are used when a large dose is needed immediately.

64. ____ By the time a transdermal patch is removed, all medication has been absorbed and there is no active ingredient left in the patch.

65. ____ The used medication patch must always be removed before a new one is applied.

66. ____ With transdermal medications, a new patch is always placed on the same site where the old patch was removed.

67. ____ Gloves are worn during the application of transdermal medications.

68. ____ The MA's initials, the date, and the time are written on a patch before it is applied.

Complete the Sentence

69. When administering medications by the rectal or vaginal routes, MAs must be especially careful to *protect patient privacy* | *remove the suppository from the foil without squashing it.*

70. If a medication is administered by the rectal or vaginal route using a(n) *applicator* | *suppository*, the device must be checked for cracks and rough edges.

71. When administering a rectal medication, the resident should be in *prone* | *Sims* position.

72. The MA should suggest that the resident *hold his breath* | *take deep breaths* to help retain the suppository.

73. Rectal suppositories are often ordered to treat constipation. Because of this, the resident may need to *drink water* | *use a bedpan or toilet* after it is administered.

74. When administering a medication by the vaginal route, the resident should be in *dorsal recumbent* | *knee-chest* position.

75. A suppository or applicator is inserted into the vagina *3–5 inches* | *3–5 centimeters.*

76. When administering medications by the rectal or vaginal route, an MA should *ask the resident's permission to continue* | *stop and report to a nurse* if the resident reports pain.

77. *Assisted living* | *Rehabilitation* facilities are more likely to give residents the option of administering their own medications.

78. When a resident administers their own medications, an MA may still assist by *placing the medications in the resident's mouth* | *checking the medication labels.*

Name: ______________________

6. Review documentation of medication administration

Fill in the Blank

1. The sixth "right" of medication administration is "right ______________."
2. An MA should never document for another ______________.
3. Resident reports of possible side effects or ______________ ______________ must be documented.
4. If an MA makes a mistake in handwritten documentation, he should not ______________ the mistake or use ______________ ______________. He should draw one line through it and write the correct information.
5. An MA must document resident ______________ of any medication and report the ______________ to the nurse.
6. When documenting, an MA should use only facility-approved terms and ______________.
7. If a nurse approves a PRN medication, most states require that the resident's ______________ to the medication be recorded in the MAR.
8. If vital sign measurements are required before a medication is administered, the measurements must be ______________ in the MAR.
9. An MA should never document ______________ completing a task.

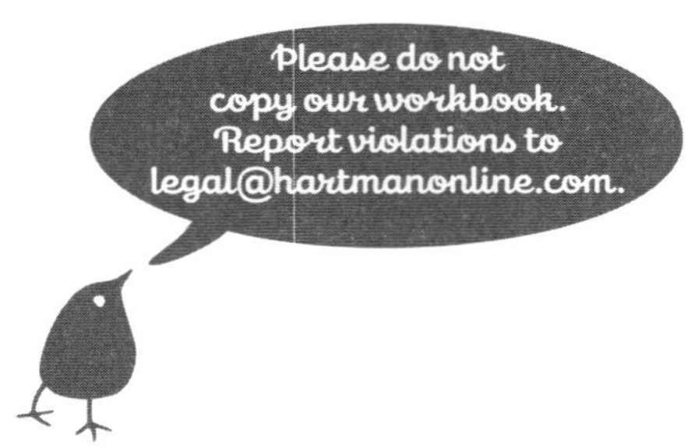

9

Preventing and Responding to Medication Errors

1. Identify common causes of medication errors

Matching

For each of the following actions by an MA, choose the letter that best matches the type of medication error the action could prevent. Letters may be used more than once.

1. _____ Before administering a medication in suspension, the MA reviews the instructions on the bottle and shakes the medication for the required amount of time.

2. _____ An MA is setting medications up for a new resident and sees a 50-mg dose on the MAR for a medication that is usually administered in a 5- or 10-mg dose. She asks the nurse about the medication; the nurse checks the provider's order and corrects the dose on the MAR to 5 mg.

3. _____ When an MA is administering a medication to a resident, the resident tells her that the pill looks different from what she has had in the past. The MA reports this to the nurse before the resident takes the medication.

4. _____ MA Douglas is setting up medications when MA Annie comes to him and asks if she can "borrow" a dose of a common medication. Douglas tells her he is sorry, but he cannot do that. He suggests that Annie talk to the nurse about getting the dose she needs.

5. _____ A resident has an order for PRN acetaminophen for headache. The nurse has assessed the resident and assigned an MA to administer the medication, but the resident tells the MA that she finds aspirin more effective. The MA says she is sorry, but that she can only administer the ordered medication.

6. _____ A resident with an order for a time-release capsule requests that the capsule be opened and the medication stirred into applesauce. The MA says she will tell the nurse if the resident is finding the capsule hard to swallow, but that this type of medication can't be opened up.

7. _____ For the past 3 days, a resident has been telling an MA that she is not feeling better, and is actually feeling worse, since she started a new medication. The MA documents her comments and reports them to the nurse every time.

8. _____ An MA keeps her facility's "Do Not Use" abbreviation list with her at all times and checks it during documentation.

(A) Failure to follow medication orders exactly

(B) Failure to follow instructions for use of a medication

(C) Failure to follow a facility's procedures and policies

(D) Failure to listen to a resident's or family member's concerns

Short Answer

9. Errors in medication administration can be dangerous, and in some cases errors in medication disposal can be dangerous as well. Why is this true for transdermal fentanyl?

____

____

____

____

____

10. Why should care be taken when using heating pads or other hot applications for a resident who has a transdermal medication applied?

____

____

____

____

11. What is a tenfold error? What is one way to help prevent these errors?

____

____

____

____

____

2. Explain steps to follow when a medication error occurs

Multiple Choice

1. In what situation(s) must medication errors be reported immediately?
   (A) Any time any medication error happens
   (B) Any time a medication error involves a drug with a black box warning
   (C) Any time a resident may be in danger as a result of the error
   (D) Any time the error was a direct result of the MA's actions

2. Which of these is an important reason to report medication errors even if they do not have a risk of resident harm?
   (A) To allow the responsible person to be punished properly
   (B) To help the facility learn and improve
   (C) To provide a legal defense in case the resident sues
   (D) To ensure errors will never happen again at the facility

3. Where are medication errors recorded?
   (A) In a resident's chart
   (B) In a resident's MAR
   (C) In a federal government database
   (D) On a general incident report or a specific medication error report

4. If a medication error is not determined to need immediate action to prevent or reduce harm, who will be responsible for assessing the resident to be sure problems do not develop?
   (A) The MA
   (B) A nursing assistant
   (C) The individual who was responsible for the error
   (D) A licensed healthcare professional

True or False

5. ____ Errors that involve OTC medications do not need to be documented.

6. ____ Setting up the wrong medication but catching the mistake before the drug is administered is an example of a *near miss*.

7. ____ Immediate firing is the usual facility response when an MA makes a medication error.

8. ____ Reporting both errors and near misses can help a facility improve its procedures related to medication safety.

Name: ______________________________

9. ____ One reason to report medication errors immediately is that some errors require immediate action to prevent or reduce resident harm.

10. ____ Although there may be consequences for healthcare workers who make medication errors, the best facility policies emphasize education and improvement of safety practices.

3. Discuss organizations involved with preventing medication errors

Fill in the Blank

1. Government and ________________________ organizations work together to reduce medication errors.
2. The Joint Commission has identified *using medications* ________________________. as one of five National Patient Safety Goals for long-term care.
3. Surveyors who inspect long-term care facilities look at rates of medication errors and classify errors as ________________________ or ________________________ ________________________.
4. Making reports on the FDA's MedWatch site is ________________________, but these reports allow the FDA to track repeated problems with the same medications.
5. Any questions a surveyor asks an MA should be answered ________________________ and ________________________.
6. The Institute for Safe Medication Practices offers materials and consulting services to ________________________ healthcare workers about medication errors.

Name: ______________________________

10

The Integumentary System and Common Medications

1. Describe the integumentary system

Complete the Sentence

1. The *largest* | *most important* organ and system in the body is the integumentary system.
2. Skin prevents injury to *bony prominences* | *internal organs*.
3. Skin also prevents the loss of too much *oxygen* | *water*, which is essential to life.
4. The skin is also a(n) *accessory* | *sense organ* that feels heat, cold, pain, touch, and pressure.
5. Blood vessels *contract* | *dilate*, or widen, when the outside temperature is too hot.
6. Blood vessels *contract* | *dilate*, or narrow, when the outside temperature is too cold.

Short Answer

Make a check mark (✓) next to normal changes of aging for the integumentary system.

7. ____ Wrinkled skin
8. ____ Swelling
9. ____ Discolored or broken skin
10. ____ Thinner, graying hair
11. ____ Less elastic skin
12. ____ Blisters, bruises, or rashes

2. Discuss common medications used to treat wounds and skin infections

Matching

Use each letter only once.

1. ____ Cellulitis
2. ____ Closed wound
3. ____ Intravenous antibiotics
4. ____ Malaise
5. ____ Methicillin-resistant *Staphylococcus aureus*
6. ____ Open wound
7. ____ Oral antibiotics

(A) A general sense of feeling unwell that may occur as a result of infection

(B) A bruise is one example

(C) May require sutures, staples, or special glue or strips

(D) Sometimes needed for severe cases of cellulitis

(E) A "super bug" that can cause complicated, hard-to-treat infections

(F) A common condition that affects the skin and soft tissue when bacteria enter

(G) Clindamycin and Bactrim are examples used to treat MRSA

Short Answer

8. What type of medication commonly ordered for cellulitis has a risk of anaphylaxis?

____

9. What are signs and symptoms of anaphylaxis?

____

____

____

10. If a resident with cellulitis has diarrhea as a side effect of antibiotic treatment, what condition should the MA observe for signs of?

____

11. What is a possible complication of cellulitis that may cause low blood pressure and fever?

____

12. Why might fluid intake and urine output be monitored for a resident taking antibiotics?

____

____

____

3. Discuss common medications used to treat dermatitis and psoriasis

True or False

1. ____ *Pruritus* is a medical term that means *inflammation.*
2. ____ *Dermatitis* is a medical term for *inflammation of the skin.*
3. ____ *Contact dermatitis, atopic dermatitis,* and *eczema* are different terms for the exact same condition.
4. ____ Hydration of the skin is very important in managing atopic dermatitis.
5. ____ Mild eczema may be treated with hydrocortisone cream.
6. ____ Antihistamines can help control an allergic response in the body.
7. ____ Immunosuppressant drugs may be ordered to treat severe cases of eczema and psoriasis.
8. ____ When applying topical corticosteroids or other topical OTC medications, MAs do not have to measure or pay attention to the amount used.
9. ____ Psoriasis is an autoimmune illness.
10. ____ Common sites for psoriasis are the feet, ears, and face.
11. ____ Exposure to possible allergens such as poison ivy and latex can cause an outbreak of psoriasis.
12. ____ Phototherapy may be used to treat psoriasis.

4. Discuss common medications used to treat fungal infections, pediculosis, and scabies

Complete the Sentence

1. A fungus is a type of *bacterium* | *living organism.*
2. Athlete's foot, or *tinea pedis,* may be prevented by use of *antifungal powder* | *mild oral antibiotics.*
3. Candidiasis of the mouth may be caused by the use of *fluoride toothpaste* | *certain medications.*
4. Untreated fungal infections of the toenails may lead to *a systemic fungal infection* | *difficulty standing and walking.*
5. Ringworm can result in a flat, circular rash anywhere on the body and is caused by *a wormlike parasite* | *a fungal infection.*
6. The common name for *pediculosis* is *lice* | *scabies.*

Short Answer

For each of the following medications or medication classes, write a condition it may be used to treat.

7. Permethrin cream

____

8. Combination of oral and topical antifungal agents

____

9. Combing/physical removal

____

10. Ivermectin (Stromectol)

____

Name: ______________________________

5. Describe burns and sunburn and response to these conditions

Multiple Choice

1. When should ointments and other topical medications be applied to burns?
    - (A) Only when they are ordered
    - (B) Immediately after any burn
    - (C) Immediately after a superficial burn
    - (D) Immediately after a partial-thickness burn as long as blisters have not yet appeared
2. Topical silver sulfadiazine is
    - (A) A prescription medication that can reduce the risk of infection and promote healing of burns
    - (B) A prescription medication that kills bacteria and reduces inflammation in an infected burn
    - (C) An OTC ointment that can protect tender skin after a superficial burn
    - (D) An OTC gel with no medicinal ingredient that cools and soothes burned skin
3. Which of the following terms describes the condition that may cause a resident taking certain medications to sunburn more easily?
    - (A) Sun susceptibility
    - (B) Burn potential
    - (C) Phototherapy
    - (D) Photosensitivity
4. In addition to sunscreen, what measures can help prevent sunburn?
    - (A) Rubbing coconut oil on the skin
    - (B) Rubbing aloe vera gel on the skin
    - (C) Wearing long sleeves and a hat
    - (D) Trying to be outside mainly during the hours of 10:00 am–2:00 pm
5. What two types of medication are in an ointment such as Cortisporin?
    - (A) Antifungal and antihistamine
    - (B) Antibiotic and corticosteroid
    - (C) Corticosteroid and analgesic
    - (D) Analgesic and antihistamine
6. What does an ointment such as Cortisporin do?
    - (A) Reduces inflammation and relieves pain
    - (B) Relieves pain and fights allergic reactions
    - (C) Reduces the chance of a fungal infection and fights allergic reactions
    - (D) Prevents infection and reduces inflammation

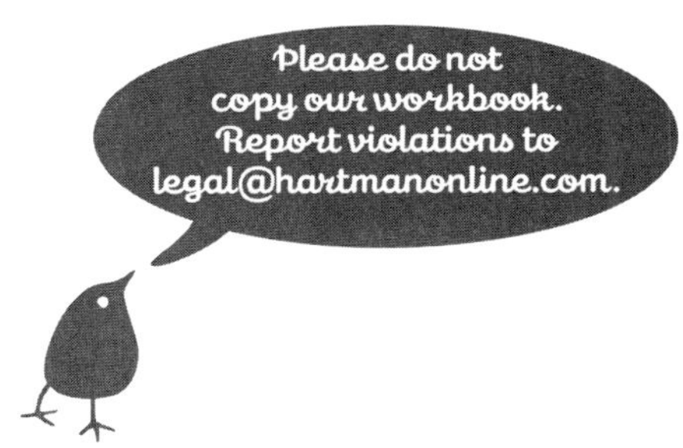

Name: ______________________________

11

The Musculoskeletal System and Common Medications

1. Describe the musculoskeletal system

True or False

1. ____ The body is shaped by muscles, bones, ligaments, tendons, and cartilage.
2. ____ The human body has 215 bones.
3. ____ Bones are made up of dead cells.
4. ____ Bones protect the body's organs.
5. ____ Muscles allow movement of body parts.
6. ____ Skeletal muscles are involuntary muscles.
7. ____ The heart is an involuntary muscle.
8. ____ One function of the musculoskeletal system is to regulate hormones in the body.

Short Answer

Make a check mark (✓) next to normal changes of aging for the musculoskeletal system.

9. ____ Muscles harden and become unable to move.
10. ____ Bones become denser and stronger.
11. ____ Body movement slows.
12. ____ Height is gradually lost.
13. ____ Osteoarthritis affects all joints.
14. ____ Muscles lose tone.

2. Discuss common medications used to treat arthritis and gout

Complete the Sentence

1. Osteoarthritis (degenerative joint disease), often affects *young adults | elderly people.*
2. Gout is a condition caused by the painful buildup of *uric acid crystals | calcium deposits* in the joints.
3. Morphine, hydromorphone, and oxycodone are all *opioid analgesics | nonsteroidal anti-inflammatory medications.*
4. One common drug that may be in multiple drugs taken by a resident is *allopurinol | acetaminophen.*
5. When a resident takes multiple drugs with the same ingredient, it is important for the provider to *not order more than the maximum daily dose from all sources | eliminate all but one source of the drug.*
6. Changes in *sleep habits | diet* may reduce levels of uric acid in the blood.

Matching

For each of the following numbered items, write as many lettered answers as apply to that item. Letters may be used more than once.

7. ________________ Acetaminophen
8. ________________ Allopurinol
9. ________________ Capsaicin cream
10. ________________ Colchicine

11. ________________ Corticosteroids

12. ________________ NSAIDs

13. ________________ Opioid analgesics

(A) Used to treat osteoarthritis

(B) Has a boxed warning related to elevated risks of myocardial infarction and stroke

(C) Reduces levels of uric acid in the body

(D) May be injected in joints affected by arthritis or gout

(E) Used to treat gout

(F) May cause bleeding in the digestive tract

(G) Used only when other treatments fail; can cause drowsiness, dizziness, and nausea, especially in elderly people

(H) Tylenol is a brand name

(I) Is a narrow therapeutic index drug

(J) Topical forms can be as effective, but with fewer side effects

(K) A cream that may be used for residents when NSAIDs are contraindicated

3. Discuss common medications used to treat osteoporosis, osteomyelitis, and back pain

Multiple Choice

1. A mineral/vitamin combination that can help prevent osteoporosis is
   (A) Magnesium/vitamin C
   (B) Calcium/vitamin C
   (C) Magnesium/vitamin D
   (D) Calcium/vitamin D

2. How do bisphosphonates work to prevent bone loss?
   (A) They act like hormones in the body.
   (B) They provide minerals the body needs to build new bone.
   (C) They slow down resorption of bone tissue.
   (D) They raise phosphorus levels in the body, which creates a hard coating on the outer layer of the bones.

3. Alendronate (Fosamax), risedronate (Actonel), and ibandronate (Boniva) are drugs that are taken
   (A) Weekly or monthly on an empty stomach with a full glass of water
   (B) Daily on an empty stomach with a full glass of water
   (C) Weekly or monthly after the evening meal with as little liquid as possible
   (D) Daily after the evening meal with as little liquid as possible

4. A broad-spectrum antibiotic is usually the first treatment for
   (A) Back pain
   (B) Osteoporosis
   (C) Osteomyelitis
   (D) Osteopenia

5. These medications, which may be ordered for back pain, can cause sedation, increasing fall risk:
   (A) Skeletal muscle relaxants
   (B) Acetaminophen
   (C) Over-the-counter NSAIDs
   (D) Prescription NSAIDs

6. Which of the following drugs has the risk of gastrointestinal tract bleeding and also may increase the risk of stroke and heart attack?
   (A) Acetaminophen
   (B) Hydromorphone
   (C) Celecoxib (Celebrex)
   (D) Tizanidine (Zanaflex)

Name: ______________________________

4. Discuss common medications used to treat strains, sprains, and fractures

Fill in the Blank

1. Strains and sprains are caused when the ______________________ ______________________ around a joint is damaged.
2. ______________________ are typically used to treat sprains and strains.
3. Both ______________________ and ______________________ medications can reduce swelling and pain from strains and sprains.
4. ______________________ such as morphine may be combined with other medications to relieve severe pain.
5. A fracture is a broken ______________________ caused by an accident or by ______________________.
6. An open fracture penetrates the ______________________ and carries a high risk of infection.
7. If surgery is required for a fracture, the patient is put under general ______________________.

   A(n) ______________________ such as vancomycin, clindamycin, or cefazolin is used to prevent infection.
8. When caring for a resident recovering from a fracture, it is important to report a change in ______________________, which could indicate infection.

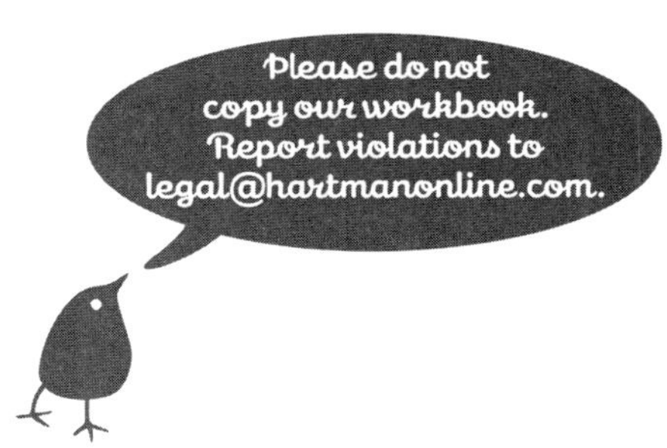

Name: ______________________________

12

The Nervous System and Common Medications

1. Describe the nervous system

Multiple Choice

1. The nervous system
   (A) Gives the body shape and structure
   (B) Controls and coordinates body functions
   (C) Is the largest organ in the body
   (D) Pumps blood through the blood vessels to the cells

2. The two main parts of the nervous system are
   (A) The cardiovascular system and the integumentary system
   (B) Neurons and receptors
   (C) The body and the brain
   (D) The central nervous system and the peripheral nervous system

3. The peripheral nervous system deals with the outer part of the body via the
   (A) Brain
   (B) Cerebrum
   (C) Nerves
   (D) Right hemisphere

4. The central nervous system is made up of
   (A) The brain and spinal cord
   (B) Muscles and bones
   (C) Neurons and receptors
   (D) The heart and lungs

Short Answer

5. List the five major sense organs of the body.

____

____

____

6. Why are the sense organs considered part of the nervous system?

____

____

____

____

____

Make a check mark (✓) by normal changes of aging to the nervous system.

7. ____ Decreased ability to move one side of the body
8. ____ Some short-term memory loss
9. ____ Vision loss that eventually results in blindness
10. ____ Slower responses and reflexes
11. ____ Difficulty speaking/forming words and understanding them
12. ____ Decreased sensitivity of nerve endings
13. ____ Inability to recognize people such as family members and regular caregivers

2. Discuss common medications used to treat cerebrovascular accident (CVA) and epilepsy

Complete the Sentence

1. A stroke occurs when the blood supply to a part of the *brain* | *heart* is blocked or a blood vessel leaks or ruptures within the *brain* | *heart*.

2. A transient ischemic attack (TIA) is a *severe type* | *warning sign* of CVA.
3. Some of the medications used to treat heart conditions are also used to prevent *seizures* | *stroke.*
4. It is very important to observe and report signs of *infection* | *bleeding* when a resident is taking antiplatelet medications.
5. The main way antiplatelet agents work is to reduce platelet *clumping* | *count,* which can prevent strokes.
6. Stroke affects the nervous system but its causes can include *integumentary* | *circulatory* system disorders.
7. The acronym *S.T.O.P.I.T.* | *B.E.F.A.S.T.* is one way to remember the sudden signs that a stroke is happening.

Short Answer

8. List five signs of bleeding to observe for in residents taking antiplatelet drugs.

____
____
____
____

9. Residents who are taking antiplatelet drugs along with other drugs that can increase bleeding risk should be observed especially carefully. List two types of drugs other than antiplatelet agents that can increase bleeding risk.

____
____

10. What is happening in the brain when a seizure occurs?

____
____

11. What are three general terms for drugs used to treat epilepsy?

____
____

12. List five possible side effects of these drugs.

____
____
____

13. Why should residents taking phenytoin (Dilantin) be observed carefully for signs of toxicity?

____
____
____

14. List three possible signs of toxicity to observe for in residents taking phenytoin (Dilantin).

____
____
____

3. Discuss common medications used to treat multiple sclerosis, myasthenia gravis, Parkinson disease, and Alzheimer disease

True or False

1. ____ For a person with myasthenia gravis, activity can make muscle weakness worse.
2. ____ Multiple sclerosis occurs when impulses from the nerves that should result in muscle movement are not transmitted properly.
3. ____ MS may be treated with drugs called immunomodulatory agents.
4. ____ There is no cure for MS, but symptoms can be treated with medications.
5. ____ Some medications for Parkinson disease replace dopamine, a neurotransmitter that is decreased by the disease.
6. ____ Side effects for cholinesterase inhibitors, a type of drug used to treat MG, are the same no matter the dose (are not dose-related).

7. ____ There are no medications that can help improve symptoms of Alzheimer disease.

8. ____ Anticholinergic drugs can reduce tremors and other involuntary movements related to Parkinson disease.

Matching

Use each letter only once.

9. ____ Anticholinergic drugs

10. ____ Cholinesterase inhibitors

11. ____ Corticosteroids

12. ____ Dopamine replacement agents

13. ____ Immunomodulatory agents

14. ____ NMDA receptor agonists

(A) May be used to treat both MS and MG; they reduce inflammation in the body and can also suppress the immune system

(B) Increase a brain chemical related to body movement that is reduced in people with Parkinson disease; side effects can include dizziness and orthostatic hypotension

(C) Reduce a brain chemical that is produced in excessive amounts in people with Alzheimer disease; can cause dizziness, headache, and constipation

(D) Block a brain chemical related to involuntary muscle movements; can reduce tremors in people with PD

(E) May be used to treat both MG and AD; they strengthen signals from the nerves to the muscles

(F) Regulate or normalize the immune system; may be used to treat MS

4. Discuss common medications used to treat pain and fatigue

Short Answer

1. Why is pain difficult to measure and observe accurately?

____

____

____

____

2. List three conditions that can cause chronic pain.

____

____

3. What type of pain, sometimes accompanied by tingling or numbness, is caused by illness or damage affecting the nervous system?

____

4. List two indications for serotonin norepinephrine reuptake inhibitors (SNRIs).

____

____

5. When might a medication such as tramadol or transdermal fentanyl be ordered for chronic pain?

____

____

____

6. List three signs to report immediately if a resident is taking an opioid medication.

____

____

____

____

7. What are three conditions that may cause neuropathic pain?

____

____

8. List four nonverbal indicators that a resident may be in pain.

____

____

____

Name: ______________________________

5. Discuss common medications used to treat mental health disorders

Fill in the Blank

1. Like physical disorders, mental health disorders produce ________________ and ________________ and can affect the body's ability to function.
2. Many medications prescribed to treat mental health conditions either block or increase the activity of different brain chemicals related to ________________.
3. Drugs used to treat mental health disorders are sometimes called ________________ medications.
4. Drugs that reduce anxiety are called ________________ drugs.
5. SSRIs and SNRIs are medications that may be ordered for anxiety or depression. When they are first administered they may increase ________________ thoughts.
6. In addition to SSRIs and SNRIs, ________________ antidepressants may be ordered to treat depression, but they can cause ________________ ________________ that include dry mouth, blurred vision, urinary retention, and constipation.
7. Drugs called mood ________________ are often prescribed to treat bipolar disorder.
8. Psychotic disorders are severe mental health disorders marked by ________________ thinking and problems with understanding ________________.
9. Schizophrenia and other psychotic disorders are treated with medications called ________________. This drug class has a boxed warning that elderly patients with ________________-related psychosis who are treated with these drugs have an increased risk of ________________.
10. Some drugs used to treat mental health disorders can cause ________________ symptoms, which involve involuntary movements such as eye spasms, twisting head, and protruding tongue.
11. Nausea, diarrhea, slurred speech, weakness, and/or confusion in a resident taking lithium for bipolar disorder could be signs of ________________.
12. SSRIs and SNRIs can cause a condition called ________________ syndrome. Shivering, diarrhea, fever, seizures, and muscle rigidity are signs of this condition.

6. Discuss common medications used to treat conditions of the sense organs

Multiple Choice

1. Glaucoma may be treated with eye drops that
   (A) Numb the eyes or dilate the pupils
   (B) Increase the flow of fluid out of the eyes or reduce the production of fluid in the eyes
   (C) Coat the eye with artificial tears
   (D) Numb the optic nerve
2. After cataract surgery a resident may be prescribed ________________ eyedrops or ointment to prevent inflammation.
   (A) NSAID
   (B) Acetaminophen
   (C) Antibiotic
   (D) Anticoagulant
3. Advanced stages of age-related macular degeneration can only be treated with
   (A) Surgery to implant an artificial lens
   (B) Medications injected into the eye
   (C) Intravenous medications
   (D) The placement of a prosthetic eye
4. In addition to promoting comfort, treatment for dry eyes
   (A) Can improve vision
   (B) May reduce intraocular pressure
   (C) May reduce the risk of infection
   (D) Can slow the development of cataracts

5. Artificial tears are used to treat dry eyes and are available
   (A) In drop and ointment forms
   (B) In drop and injection forms
   (C) In ointment and spray forms
   (D) In injection and cream forms

6. What infection prevention measures must be used when a resident has conjunctivitis?
   (A) Standard Precautions only
   (B) Standard Precautions and Airborne Precautions
   (C) Standard Precautions and Droplet Precautions
   (D) Standard Precautions and Contact Precautions

Short Answer

7. What is the common name for the condition *acute otitis media*?

____

8. What are two classes of medications that may be used to treat acute otitis media?

____

____

9. What do *cerumenolytics* do?

____

____

10. Why should an MA never insert a swab or other object in a resident's ear to remove ear wax?

____

____

____

Name: ______________________________

13

The Circulatory System and Common Medications

1. Describe the circulatory system

Multiple Choice

1. What functions as the pump of the circulatory system?
   (A) The heart
   (B) The lungs
   (C) Lymph fluid
   (D) Blood

2. What do platelets do?
   (A) They defend the body against foreign substances.
   (B) They cause the blood to clot after an injury.
   (C) They carry oxygen to all parts of the body.
   (D) They allow red blood cells to carry iron.

3. Which of these choices is the most complete list of the parts of the circulatory system?
   (A) The lungs, the heart, and breathing passages
   (B) Red blood cells, white blood cells, and platelets
   (C) The heart, blood vessels, and blood
   (D) Capillaries, arteries, and veins

4. Oxygen is carried from the lungs to all parts of the body by
   (A) Lymphocytes
   (B) Thrombocytes
   (C) Leukocytes
   (D) Erythrocytes

Short Answer

Make a check mark (✓) by normal changes of aging to the circulatory system.

5. ____ The heart valves stop working
6. ____ The heart beats faster
7. ____ Blood flow decreases
8. ____ Blood clots more quickly
9. ____ Blood pressure decreases
10. ____ Blood vessels narrow
11. ____ The heart pumps less efficiently
12. ____ Capacity for exercise increases

2. Discuss common medications used to treat hypertension

Matching

Use each letter only once.

1. ____ Angiotensin-converting enzyme (ACE) inhibitors
2. ____ Angiotensin receptor blockers (ARBs)
3. ____ Beta adrenergic blocking agents (beta-blockers)
4. ____ Calcium channel blockers
5. ____ Diuretics
6. ____ Potassium-sparing diuretics
7. ____ Thiazide diuretics
8. ____ Vasodilators

(A) General term for drugs that control blood pressure by reducing the amount of fluid in the body; sometimes called *water pills*

(B) One type of drug that blocks chemicals that increase blood pressure; generic names end in *-sartan*

(C) Drugs that relax the heart and blood vessels, lowering blood pressure; generic names end in *-pine*

(D) Drugs that reduce the amount of fluid in the body without reducing the levels of an important mineral

(E) One type of drug that affects the action of chemicals that increase blood pressure; angioedema is a rare but dangerous adverse effect; generic names end in *-pril*

(F) Drugs that reduce blood pressure by widening blood vessels in the body

(G) One type of drug that blocks chemicals that increase blood pressure; these drugs may also reduce heart rate; generic names end in *-olol*

(H) A stronger type of drug that reduces the amount of fluid in the body

Fill in the Blank

9. Diuretics increase the need to ____________________. These medications are usually administered in the ____________________ to avoid sleep disturbance.

10. Monitor blood pressure and pulse as directed. ____________________ can result from taking these drugs. This may increase the risk of falls.

11. It is important to carefully observe residents with diabetes who also take beta-blockers because side effects of beta-blockers are similar to symptoms of ____________________ blood sugar. ____________________, fainting, loss of balance, and fatigue should be reported to the nurse immediately.

12. Angioedema causes ____________________ of the lips and tongue.

3. Discuss common medications used to treat coronary artery disease and related conditions

Complete the Sentence

1. Cholesterol is a *fat-like* | *infection-fighting* substance in the blood.
2. Too much LDL cholesterol in the blood can lead to buildup in the *chambers of the heart* | *arteries.*
3. Hypercholesterolemia is the medical term for *low* | *high* cholesterol.
4. The drugs most often used to control cholesterol levels are called *statins* | *beta-blockers.*
5. At higher doses, these same drugs may be used to treat *coronary artery disease* | *hypertension.*
6. *ACE inhibitors* | *Antiplatelet drugs* are often ordered for people with CAD to prevent clots from forming in narrowed arteries.
7. When nitroglycerin is used before activities that might cause chest pain, it is being used *prophylactically* | *responsively.*
8. After a heart attack, low-dose *acetaminophen* | *aspirin* may be given on a continuing basis.

Multiple Choice

9. This type of medication disrupts the body's fat-absorbing process, which lowers the amount of fat in the blood:
(A) Statins
(B) Vasodilators
(C) Bile acid sequestrants
(D) Antiplatelet agents

10. Residents with high cholesterol may have provider orders to take supplements for their condition, including
(A) Niacin and fish oil
(B) Magnesium and melatonin
(C) Vitamin D and calcium
(D) Zinc and vitamin C

11. Drugs often used after a heart attack include medications that may also be used for
    (A) Asthma and chronic obstructive pulmonary disease
    (B) Hypertension and hypercholesterolemia
    (C) Depression and anxiety
    (D) Chronic pain and osteoarthritis

12. These drugs may be contraindicated for residents who have had an MI:
    (A) Beta-blockers
    (B) Anticoagulants
    (C) Antiplatelet agents
    (D) Nonsteroidal anti-inflammatory drugs

4. Discuss common medications used to treat heart failure and dysrhythmia

True or False

1. ____ Digoxin is a narrow therapeutic index drug that may be ordered for heart failure or dysrhythmia.
2. ____ Most drugs used to treat heart failure are never used for other circulatory system disorders.
3. ____ Loop diuretics are weaker than other types of diuretics.
4. ____ Some drugs for heart failure dilate both arteries and veins, reducing the heart's workload
5. ____ One of the risks of atrial fibrillation is that it can lead to stroke.
6. ____ Some medications used to treat hypertension are also used to treat dysrhythmias.

Short Answer

7. What risk is increased if a resident takes both loop diuretics and NSAIDs?

____

8. List three conditions that may contribute to heart failure.

____

____

9. What effects of digoxin make it useful in treating heart failure?

____

____

10. What side effects should an MA observe for and report when a resident is taking digoxin?

____

____

____

5. Discuss common medications used to treat conditions related to the blood

Matching

Use each letter only once.

1. ____ Acetaminophen
2. ____ Antiplatelet agents
3. ____ Direct oral anticoagulant
4. ____ NSAIDs
5. ____ Oral iron
6. ____ Warfarin

(A) Analgesics contraindicated for residents who take anticoagulants

(B) Does not require regular blood testing or consistent vitamin K intake

(C) Requires regular blood testing and consistent vitamin K intake

(D) Used to treat a form of anemia; may cause constipation

(E) Used to treat the pain related to phlebitis if other drugs are contraindicated

(F) Used to prevent arterial clots caused when blood pools in the heart

Name: ______________________________

Complete the Sentence

7. When administering oral iron, it is important to know that many foods *prevent or slow* | *increase or speed* its absorption.

8. Falls, especially falls that cause head injury, are dangerous in residents who are taking anticoagulant medications due to the risk of *severe head pain* | *intracranial bleeding.*

9. *Nosebleeds and bruising* | *vomiting and diarrhea* are signs that may indicate excessive bleeding in a resident taking anticoagulants.

10. Vitamin K is necessary for the formation of *blood clots* | *hemoglobin.*

11. Iron is necessary for the formation of *blood clots* | *hemoglobin.*

12. Blood circulates through the body, delivering *oxygen* | *carbon dioxide* and nutrients and removing *oxygen* | *carbon dioxide* and waste products.

14

The Respiratory System and Common Medications

1. Describe the respiratory system

True or False

1. ____ Respiration occurs in the lungs.
2. ____ Expiration is breathing in.
3. ____ The respiratory system brings oxygen into the body and eliminates carbon dioxide produced as the body uses oxygen.

Short Answer

Make a check mark (✓) by normal changes of aging to the respiratory system.

4. ____ Lung capacity decreases
5. ____ Blood oxygen level increases
6. ____ Lung strength decreases
7. ____ Voice is eventually lost completely
8. ____ Breathing deepens

2. Discuss common medications used to treat rhinitis, sinusitis, and asthma

Multiple Choice

1. Allergic rhinitis may be accompanied by other allergy symptoms such as
   (A) High fever
   (B) Red, itchy, watery eyes
   (C) Body aches
   (D) Peripheral edema
2. Most cases of sinusitis are not helped by
   (A) The use of antibiotics
   (B) Rest and fluids
   (C) The use of decongestants
   (D) The use of saline
3. Most residents who have asthma will have these two types of asthma medication ordered:
   (A) A decongestant and bronchodilator
   (B) An oral medication and a nasal spray
   (C) A nebulized medication and disc-style inhaler
   (D) A maintenance medication and a rescue medication
4. Inhaled corticosteroids are a type of
   (A) Fast-acting bronchodilator
   (B) Long-acting bronchodilator
   (C) Medication used to make asthma flare-ups less likely
   (D) Medication used to treat an asthma attack as it is happening
5. Which of the following is true of oral corticosteroids?
   (A) They are taken daily by most residents with asthma.
   (B) They are administered by nebulizer.
   (C) They clear mucus from the lungs.
   (D) A short course may be ordered to bring asthma under control.

True or False

6. ____ A resident should blow their nose immediately after a medication is administered by nasal spray.
7. ____ A high fever and severe symptoms in a resident with sinusitis should be reported to the nurse.
8. ____ Metered dose inhalers should be gently turned upside down and then right side up again one time before they are administered.

Name: ______________________________

9. ____ Strong odors and strenuous exercise can trigger asthma attacks in some residents.

10. ____ Residents should rinse their mouths after an inhaled corticosteroid is administered.

3. Discuss common medications used to treat influenza, COVID-19, bronchitis, and pneumonia

Fill in the Blank

1. Influenza can be dangerous for residents because it may lead to ______________________ or to inflammation of tissues in the ______________________ or ______________________.

2. One way to protect residents against influenza is for residents and their caregivers to be ______________________ each year.

3. Respiratory ______________________ is a serious risk when COVID-19 causes severe disease.

4. ______________________ medications can reduce the severity of influenza and COVID-19 illnesses.

5. Pneumonia is an illness that can be caused by a ______________________, ______________________, or ______________________ infection.

6. ______________________ agents are drugs used to control a cough.

7. A medication that thins out mucus in the lungs, making it easier to cough out, is a(n) ______________________.

8. COVID-19 is a disease spread by ______________________ particles and ______________________ droplets.

9. Influenza or cold viruses can cause ______________________ when they cause irritation and inflammation of the lining of the bronchi.

10. A high fever, chills, cough, greenish or yellow sputum, chest pains, and a rapid pulse are signs and symptoms of ______________________.

11. The type of medication used to treat pneumonia may depend on whether the pneumonia was acquired at a(n) ______________________.

Short Answer

12. Why is it important to pay attention to the amounts of all active ingredients when administering OTC medications for cold, flu, or COVID-19 symptoms?

____

____

____

____

13. OTC decongestants may be contraindicated for some residents with a common condition. What is that condition and why might decongestants be contraindicated?

____

____

____

____

14. How should residents be positioned to take oral medications? What respiratory condition may be prevented in this way?

____

____

____

____

4. Discuss common medications used to treat chronic obstructive pulmonary disease (COPD)

Complete the Sentence

1. Residents with COPD have trouble breathing, especially with getting air *into* | *out of* their lungs.
2. Treatment for chronic bronchitis includes stopping smoking and *possibly* | *inhaled, oral, and injected* medications.
3. There are two chronic lung diseases that are grouped under COPD: chronic bronchitis and *pneumonia* | *emphysema.*
4. Medications for COPD include bronchodilators and drugs that reduce *oxygen levels* | *inflammation in the lungs.*
5. The effectiveness of inhaled medications depends on *proper administration* | *the temperature of the room.*

5. Discuss common medications used to treat pleurisy, atelectasis, and pulmonary embolism (PE)

Multiple Choice

1. Pulmonary embolism is usually caused by blood clots that have traveled to the
   (A) Heart from superficial veins in the limbs
   (B) Lungs from superficial veins in the limbs
   (C) Brain from deep veins in the limbs
   (D) Lungs from deep veins in the limbs
2. Treatment for PE usually includes medications to
   (A) Dissolve clots and prevent new clots from forming
   (B) Open the airways and increase circulation
   (C) Reduce anxiety and promote rest
   (D) Increase clotting and prevent blood loss
3. In addition to treating any underlying cause of pleurisy, medication may include this type of medication to control pain:
   (A) Mucolytic
   (B) Anxiolytic
   (C) Analgesic
   (D) Antitussive
4. Atelectasis caused by excessive mucus in the lungs is a possible complication of
   (A) Pneumonia
   (B) Seasonal allergies
   (C) Hypertension
   (D) Intense exercise
5. Inflammation of the layers of tissue that separate the lungs from the chest wall is called
   (A) Asthma
   (B) Pulmonary edema
   (C) Collapsed lung
   (D) Pleurisy
6. Treatment for pneumothorax may include
   (A) Insertion of tubes to remove air from the chest cavity
   (B) Insertion of tubes to pump air into the chest cavity
   (C) Placement of the resident in a sealed, pressurized oxygen chamber
   (D) Administration of anticoagulant medications

6. Discuss common medications used to treat tuberculosis (TB)

True or False

1. ____ A combination of several antiviral medications is used to treat TB.
2. ____ There are two phases to TB treatment: the intensive phase and the continuation phase.
3. ____ Medications given for TB have few side effects and no known adverse effects.

Name: ______________________________

4. ____ A person who has TB but is improving quickly can stop taking medications.

5. ____ When bacteria cannot be killed by a drug, they are considered *resistant* to that drug.

6. ____ Multidrug-resistant TB is easier to treat than other forms of TB.

7. ____ People with compromised immune systems are more likely to get TB than other people.

8. ____ Tuberculosis is not very contagious; Standard Precautions are enough to prevent its spread.

9. ____ Whether a resident with TB is placed in an airborne infection isolation room or not depends on the resident's preference.

10. ____ Failure to take TB medications as ordered is a major factor in the spread of TB.

15

The Urinary System and Common Medications

1. Describe the urinary system

Short Answer

1. List the two vital functions of the urinary system.

_____

_____

_____

_____

_____

2. What are the parts of the urinary system?

_____

_____

_____

_____

_____

Make a check mark (✓) by normal changes of aging to the urinary system.

3. ____ The kidneys fail.
4. ____ The bladder cannot hold urine effectively, causing urinary incontinence.
5. ____ Bladder muscle tone weakens.
6. ____ The kidneys filter blood more efficiently.
7. ____ The bladder holds less urine, causing frequent urination.
8. ____ The bladder may not empty completely, causing a greater risk of infection.

2. Discuss common medications used to treat urinary incontinence

Complete the Sentence

1. Before medications are used to treat urinary incontinence, residents' *dietary habits* | *fluid intake* may be reviewed.
2. Incontinence *is* | *is not* a normal change of aging.
3. One type of *antidepressant* | *antihypertensive* medication has been shown to help incontinence.
4. *Antispasmodic agents* | *Estrogen* may be administered vaginally to treat incontinence.
5. Urinary incontinence is a major risk factor for *pressure injuries* | *falls*.
6. Incontinence pads or briefs *should* | *should not* be referred to as diapers.
7. In female residents, exercises that strengthen the muscles in the *lower abdomen* | *pelvic floor* can help prevent incontinence.

3. Discuss common medications used to treat urinary retention and urinary obstruction

Multiple Choice

1. Urinary obstruction may be caused by
   (A) Kidney stones
   (B) Excessive fluid intake
   (C) Normal changes of aging
   (D) High blood pressure

2. Which of the following is true of urinary retention?
   (A) It tends to improve without treatment.
   (B) It is not associated with any other health risks.
   (C) It is more common in women.
   (D) It is more common in men.

Matching

For each of the following numbered items, write as many lettered answers as apply to that item. Letters may be used more than once.

3. ____________ Alpha-blocking agents
4. ____________ Benign prostatic hyperplasia
5. ____________ Cholinergic agents
6. ____________ Urinary obstruction
7. ____________ Chronic urinary retention

(A) May cause orthostatic hypotension and dizziness

(B) May be caused by kidney stones

(C) One part of treatment may be increasing fluid intake

(D) Sometimes treated with different drugs in men and women

(E) Increase the contraction of the bladder muscle

(F) A urinary condition more common in men

(G) May cause urinary retention in men

(H) Relax the prostate and bladder in men and the bladder in women

(I) Can cause excessive salivation, nausea, diarrhea, or abdominal cramps

4. Discuss common medications used to treat urinary tract infection (UTI)

True or False

1. _____ *Cystitis* is the medical term for inflammation of the bladder.
2. _____ Sepsis is a possible complication of UTI.
3. _____ Phenazopyridine is a medication that does not cure a bladder infection, but may reduce pain.
4. _____ Urinary tract infections are usually caused by fungi.
5. _____ UTI is more common in women, in part because the urethra is shorter in females than in males and pathogens can reach the bladder more easily.
6. _____ The antibiotic used to treat a UTI depends on where the infection is and how severe it is.
7. _____ Intravenous antibiotics may be used to treat some UTIs.
8. _____ Fluid intake should be discouraged when a resident has a UTI.
9. _____ Fever, chills, nausea/vomiting, and flank pain may be signs and symptoms of a bladder infection moving to the kidneys.
10. _____ Confusion is a rare symptom of UTI in elderly people.

5. Discuss common medications used to treat kidney disease and fluid imbalance

Multiple Choice

1. This condition may contribute to chronic kidney disease (CKD):
   (A) Diabetes
   (B) Asthma
   (C) Rheumatoid arthritis
   (D) Cardiac dysrhythmia

2. Which of the following conditions is often seen together with CKD?
   (A) Dermatitis
   (B) Respiratory failure
   (C) Hypertension
   (D) Stroke

Name: ______________________________

3. Classes of medications often ordered for residents with CKD include
   (A) Antiarrythmics, diuretics, and cholinergic agents
   (B) Diuretics, anxiolytics, and anticoagulants
   (C) Antiplatelet agents, beta-blockers, and NSAIDs
   (D) ACE inhibitors, angiotensin receptor blockers, and diuretics

4. Why might a resident with CKD take a statin medication?
   (A) To reduce blood pressure
   (B) To reduce lipids (fats) in the bloodstream
   (C) To regulate heart rate and rhythm
   (D) To reduce edema (swelling)

Fill in the Blank

5. Because the kidneys filter waste from the blood, kidney disease can affect the entire ____________________. It is a complex syndrome that involves multiple ____________________.

6. ____________________ and ____________________ are some of the conditions that can cause dehydration.

7. Severe dehydration is treated with ____________________ fluids, often in a hospital setting.

8. MAs should know residents' mental and physical ____________________ (their personal "normal"). They should report ____________________ to the nurse.

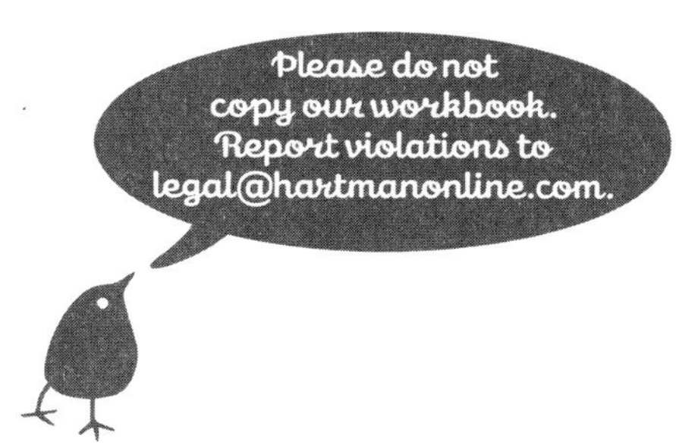

Name: ______________________________

Name: ______________________________

16

The Gastrointestinal System and Common Medications

1. Describe the gastrointestinal system

Crossword

Across

1. This type of organ is not part of the gastrointestinal tract but helps to prepare food so that it can be absorbed
2. Process of expelling wastes (made up of the waste products of food and fluids) that are not absorbed into the cells

Down

3. Semisolid material made up of water, solid waste material, bacteria, and mucus that passes through the rectum and out of the body
4. Transfer of nutrients from the intestines to the cells
5. Process of preparing food physically and chemically so that it can be absorbed into the cells
6. Another name for the gastrointestinal system is the ______________________ system.
7. Food passes through this part of the gastrointestinal tract first

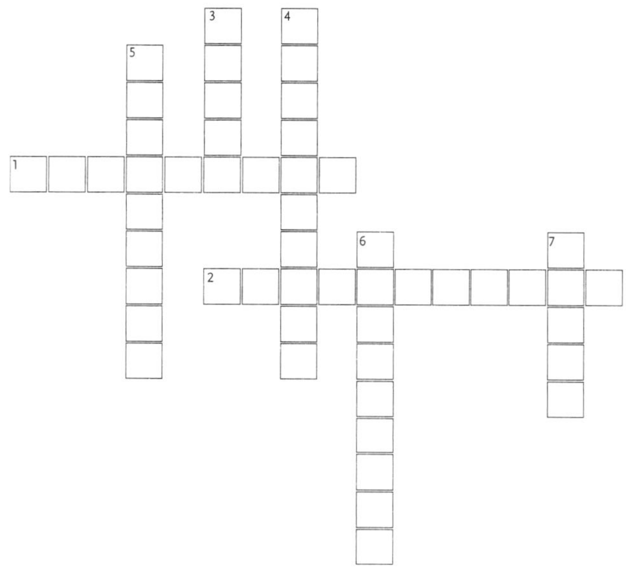

Short Answer

Make a check mark (✓) by normal changes of aging to the gastrointestinal system.

8. ____ The process of digestion gets faster.
9. ____ Diarrhea occurs more often due to the increased speed of digestion.
10. ____ Decreased saliva production affects the ability to chew and swallow.
11. ____ Dulled sense of taste may result in poor appetite.
12. ____ Digestion is less efficient.
13. ____ Vitamin and mineral absorption improves, which means fewer vitamins and minerals need to be consumed.

2. Discuss common medications used to treat stomatitis and ulcerative gingivitis

Complete the Sentence

1. Using a toothbrush with *hard* | *soft bristles* can cause mouth pain and irritation.
2. *Failure to use* | *Poorly fitted* dentures can also cause stomatitis.
3. Treatment of stomatitis may include the use of *topical* | *inhaled* anesthetics, corticosteroids, antibiotics, or antifungal agents.
4. Ulcerative gingivitis is also called acute *inflammatory* | *necrotizing* ulcerative gingivitis.
5. Initial treatment for ulcerative gingivitis is a thorough cleaning performed by an oral hygienist or *dentist* | *registered nurse.*
6. Regular rinses with a mouthwash containing *chlorhexidine* | *isopropyl alcohol* or with diluted hydrogen peroxide are part of the treatment for ulcerative gingivitis.
7. Irritation or inflammation in the mouth can be made worse by *sweet* | *acidic* or spicy foods.
8. *Corticosteroids* | *Antifungals* can cause oral candidiasis.
9. Residents who are cognitively impaired may have topical agents applied with a swab to prevent the resident from *swallowing* | *spitting out* the medication.
10. One example of a systemic symptom that may indicate an infection in the mouth has spread in the body is *discoloration of the gums* | *malaise.*

3. Discuss common medications used to treat gastroesophageal reflux disease (GERD), peptic ulcer disease, and gastritis

Short Answer

1. What are two classes of medication often used to treat GERD? What are the endings of generic drug names for each class?

____

____

____

____

2. How does each of these medication classes limit the amount of acid in the stomach?

____

____

____

____

3. Why might an antibiotic be ordered to treat ulcers? What other type of medication is ordered along with the antibiotic in these cases?

____

____

____

____

____

4. What is gastritis? Why might elderly people be more likely than younger people to have gastritis?

____

____

____

____

True or False

5. _____ Proton pump inhibitors should be administered 30–60 minutes before a meal.

6. _____ Diet and lifestyle changes can help control GERD.

7. _____ NSAIDs are the preferred painkillers for residents with peptic ulcer disease.

8. _____ Dairy products such as lowfat milk usually increase ulcer pain.

9. _____ Antacids can relieve gastrointestinal pain immediately, but other medications for these conditions can take time to work.

10. _____ Citrus fruits and beverages, tomatoes, chocolate, fatty foods, spicy foods, caffeine, and alcohol can all worsen GERD or ulcer pain.

11. _____ Residents with GERD should lie down and rest immediately after each meal.

12. _____ Peptic ulcers can cause bleeding which can result in stools that appear black and tarry.

4. Discuss common medications used to treat nausea, vomiting, diarrhea, and gastroenteritis

Multiple Choice

1. Drugs that relieve nausea and slow or prevent vomiting are called
   (A) Antimotility agents
   (B) Laxatives
   (C) Antiemetics
   (D) Bile acid sequestrants

2. To prevent dehydration caused by vomiting or diarrhea, rehydration beverages containing these substances may be ordered:
   (A) Electrolytes and glucose
   (B) Caffeine and electrolytes
   (C) Glucose and beneficial bacteria
   (D) Beneficial bacteria and lowfat milk

3. If a resident who is vomiting often cannot take an oral tablet to slow vomiting, the medication may be ordered as a(n)
   (A) Transdermal patch
   (B) Oral liquid
   (C) Chewable tablet
   (D) Enteric-coated tablet

4. Treatments for diarrhea include
   (A) Antiemetic agents and rehydration fluids
   (B) H2 blockers and probiotics
   (C) Antacids and antimotility agents
   (D) Antimotility agents and probiotics

5. Although it is often called *stomach flu*, ______________________ is the medical term for irritation or inflammation of the digestive tract usually caused by norovirus or rotavirus.
   (A) Influenza A
   (B) Influenza B
   (C) Gastroenteritis
   (D) Peritonitis

Fill in the Blank

6. Signs of dehydration that must be reported to the nurse include dry mouth/lips, ______________________ eyes, dark or strong-smelling urine, and ______________________.

7. An MA should report to the nurse immediately if a resident cannot ______________________ an oral medication or ______________________ immediately after taking a medication.

8. The viruses that cause ______________________ are highly contagious. MAs should ______________________ frequently with soap and water.

9. Chronic watery diarrhea may be caused by a spore-forming bacterium called *C. difficile*. Alcohol-based ______________________ is not effective against *C. difficile*.

5. Discuss common medications used to treat constipation and hemorrhoids

True or False

1. ____ The first line of treatment for hemorrhoids is to reduce fluid intake.
2. ____ Constipation can cause abdominal swelling, gas, and irritability.
3. ____ Topical hydrocortisone and anesthetics are commonly used to treat hemorrhoids.
4. ____ One way that laxatives can work is by increasing the movement of the intestines.
5. ____ Laxatives administered rectally work more slowly than oral laxatives.
6. ____ Increasing fiber intake may be part of the first line of treatment for both constipation and hemorrhoids.
7. ____ Constipation is the only condition that may be treated with stool softeners.
8. ____ A resident who is constipated should be encouraged to strain as much as needed to have a bowel movement.
9. ____ An MA should not administer a laxative to a resident with diarrhea without first reporting to the nurse.
10. ____ Inactivity and aging are risk factors for constipation.

6. Discuss common medications used to treat conditions affecting the bowels

Matching

Use each letter only once.

1. ____ Crohn disease
2. ____ Diverticulitis
3. ____ Inflammatory bowel disease (IBD)
4. ____ Irritable bowel syndrome (IBS)
5. ____ Peritonitis
6. ____ Ulcerative colitis

(A) A medical emergency that can occur as a complication of diverticulitis

(B) A form of IBD that affects a continuous area of the gastrointestinal system; treatment includes immunosuppressants and medications, such as corticosteroids, to reduce inflammation

(C) A condition that relates to bowel function and may cause diarrhea, constipation, or both on a regular basis; treatment is based on symptoms and may include antispasmodic agents to reduce cramping

(D) A term for conditions in which the bowel is chronically inflamed; these conditions cause physical damage to the gastrointestinal tract

(E) A condition caused by inflammation of small pouches in the colon; treated with oral or IV antibiotics

(F) A form of IBD that most commonly affects the small intestine and can cause inflammation in patches, among healthy tissue; treatment includes immunosuppressants and medications, such as corticosteroids, to reduce inflammation

7. Discuss common medications used to treat conditions affecting the liver, gallbladder, and pancreas

Short Answer

1. In general terms, what part do the liver, gallbladder, and pancreas play in digestion?

____

____

____

2. List four possible causes of hepatitis.

____

____

____

____

Name: ______________________________

3. Which forms of hepatitis are considered bloodborne diseases?

____

____

4. Hepatitis A is vaccine preventable. Which other form of hepatitis can be prevented by vaccine?

____

5. What class of medications can help fight hepatitis and prevent it from damaging the liver?

____

Fill in the Blank

6. ____________________ and chronic alcoholism are common causes of cirrhosis, a liver disease in which liver tissue is replaced with ______________________ tissue.

7. If cirrhosis causes gastrointestinal bleeding, a short course of ______________________ may be ordered to prevent infection.

8. Repeated cases of acute pancreatitis can lead to ______________________ pancreatitis.

9. Pancreatitis can cause severe pain that is often treated with acetaminophen and the ______________________ analgesics codeine and morphine. ______________________ are not used due to increased ulcer and bleeding risks.

10. Medications used to dissolve gallstones may take ______________________ ______________________ to dissolve the stones. Diarrhea, constipation, stomach upset, ______________________, and headache are common side effects.

11. If a resident is taking ursodiol or chenodiol for cholelithiasis, blood may be tested regularly. This is because these drugs can affect ______________________ function.

12. Residents with pancreatitis may take ______________________ for extended periods. MAs must be aware of all ordered medications containing this drug. Because of the extended use, the maximum daily dose may be lowered to ______________________ milligrams.

Name: ____________________

17

The Endocrine System and Common Medications

1. Describe the endocrine system

True or False

1. ____ One function of the endocrine system is to maintain blood sugar levels.
2. ____ Decreased insulin production is a normal change of aging.
3. ____ Glands are organs that produce red and white blood cells.
4. ____ The endocrine system is made of nodes and vessels that store and circulate disease-fighting fluids throughout the body.
5. ____ The endocrine system influences growth and development.
6. ____ With age, the body becomes less able to handle stress.
7. ____ Regulating metabolism and maintaining homeostasis are functions of the endocrine system.
8. ____ Levels of hormones, such as estrogen and progesterone, increase with age.

2. Discuss common medications used to treat diabetes

Matching

Use each letter only once.

1. ____ Blood glucose testing
2. ____ HbA1c
3. ____ Insulin
4. ____ Insulin for inhalation
5. ____ Insulin resistance
6. ____ Oral antidiabetic drugs
7. ____ Type 1 diabetes
8. ____ Type 2 diabetes

(A) Medications that decrease glucose production and/or absorption, increase the release of insulin, or increase the body's sensitivity to insulin

(B) Contraindicated for people with asthma or COPD

(C) Often develops after age 35; can usually be controlled with diet and/or oral medications

(D) A hormone that works to remove natural sugar from the blood and into the cells for energy for the body; may be administered as a medication to residents with diabetes

(E) A measurement of average glucose levels over a 2- to 3-month period

(F) Usually diagnosed in children and young adults; must be treated with insulin and a special diet

(G) Situation in which the body fails to properly use insulin

(H) Must be done regularly for residents with diabetes

Complete the Sentence

9. Metformin and glipizide are antidiabetic drugs that are administered *orally | by subcutaneous injection*.
10. A(n) *intravenous | fingerstick* blood glucose test is a common test performed often on residents with diabetes.

11. Hypoglycemia is a complication of diabetes that can result from *too much* | *too little* insulin or *too much* | *too little* food.

12. A resident experiencing hypoglycemia needs to receive *insulin* | *glucose* immediately.

13. Diabetic ketoacidosis (DKA) is a dangerous complication caused by having *too much* | *too little* insulin in the body.

14. Most types of insulin are administered by *mouth* | *subcutaneous injection.*

15. Reduced circulation in residents with diabetes can lead to *rapid* | *poor* wound healing.

16. Injectable antidiabetic drugs such as semaglutide and tirzepatide promote weight loss and may reduce the risk of *asthma* | *cardiovascular disease.*

3. Discuss common medications used to treat thyroid disorders

Multiple Choice

1. How does radioactive iodine work to treat hyperthyroidism?
   (A) It increases the ability of the thyroid gland to produce thyroid hormone.
   (B) It lowers the ability of the thyroid gland to produce thyroid hormone.
   (C) It causes the thyroid gland to grow, allowing a provider to observe it more easily.
   (D) It completely dissolves the thyroid gland.

2. Thyroid replacement therapy involves
   (A) Administering oral medications that replace thyroid hormone in people with hypothyroidism
   (B) Administering oral medications that replace thyroid hormone in people with hyperthyroidism
   (C) Transplanting a healthy thyroid gland into a person whose thyroid gland is not working correctly
   (D) Replacing thyroid hormones in the body with intravenous infusions of different hormones

3. Surgical removal of part of the thyroid gland is a possible treatment for
   (A) Diabetes
   (B) Hyperglycemia
   (C) Hypothyroidism
   (D) Hyperthyroidism

4. The drugs methimazole and propylthiouracil slow the production of thyroid hormone. Residents who take these drugs will have their blood tested regularly to
   (A) Monitor liver function and measure thyroid levels
   (B) Measure thyroid levels only
   (C) Monitor liver function only
   (D) Monitor blood count

5. In a resident with hypothyroidism who takes a thyroid hormone replacement, increased heart rate, palpitation, weight loss, and irritability are signs that the resident's
   (A) Hypothyroidism is getting worse
   (B) Thyroid gland has become overactive
   (C) Dose of thyroid hormone is too low
   (D) Dose of thyroid hormone is too high

6. Thyroid hormone replacement medications must be administered
   (A) With a full glass of milk
   (B) With a soft food such as applesauce or pudding
   (C) On an empty stomach
   (D) After a complete meal

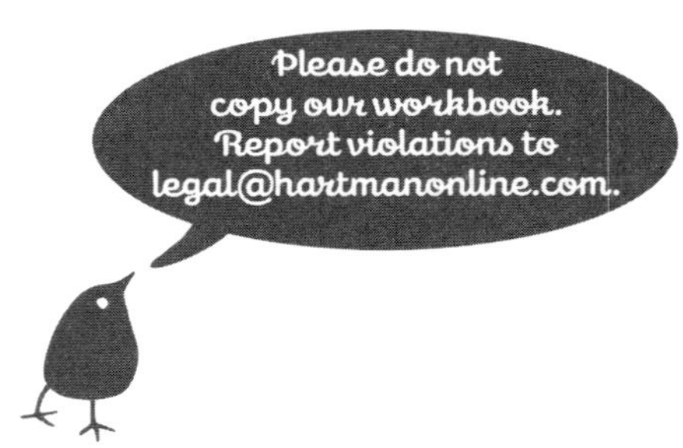

18

The Reproductive System and Common Medications

1. Describe the reproductive system

Fill in the Blank

1. The reproductive system allows human beings to reproduce, or create new ________________________________.
2. Reproduction begins when a male's and female's sex cells (________________________ and ________________________) join.
3. For males, the function of the reproductive system is to manufacture sperm and the male hormone ________________________.
4. In addition to producing sex cells and hormones, the female reproductive system provides an environment for the development of a ________________________.

Short Answer

Make a check mark (✓) next to normal changes of aging for the reproductive system.

5. ____ Menstrual periods that become heavier and longer
6. ____ Development of prostate cancer
7. ____ A decrease in estrogen, which leads to a loss of calcium
8. ____ Erectile dysfunction
9. ____ Decreased sperm production
10. ____ Vaginal walls become drier and thinner
11. ____ Enlargement of the prostate gland

2. Discuss common medications used to treat conditions of the male reproductive system

Matching

Use each letter only once.

1. ____ Alpha-blockers
2. ____ Nitrates (such as nitroglycerin)
3. ____ Prostate-specific antigen (PSA)
4. ____ Sildenafil (Viagra) and vardenafil (Staxyn)
5. ____ Tadalafil (Cialis)

(A) Used to treat erectile dysfunction (ED)

(B) Rising levels in the blood can be a sign of prostate cancer

(C) Generic names end with *-osin*; used to treat benign prostatic hyperplasia (BPH)

(D) Should not be taken with medications used to treat ED; can cause a sudden drop in blood pressure

(E) Used to treat BPH and ED

Short Answer

6. What form of reproductive system cancer is common in older men?

____

7. What happens to the prostate gland in BPH?

____

____

____

8. What are three possible complications of BPH?

____

____

____

____

____

9. What are the most common physical causes of ED?

____

____

3. Discuss common medications used to treat conditions of the female reproductive system

Complete the Sentence

1. Many conditions relate to or may be made *better* | *worse* by hormonal changes after menopause.
2. Vaginal dryness and thinning of the vaginal walls can increase the risk of urinary tract infection and *osteoporosis* | *vaginitis*.
3. Hormone replacement therapy may be ordered when a woman is at high risk for *osteoporosis* | *bacterial vaginosis*.
4. Miconazole, tioconazole, and fluconazole are all common *antibiotics* | *fungicides* that can effectively treat yeast infections.
5. Bacterial vaginosis may be treated with medications administered orally or *by injection* | *vaginally*.
6. Vaginal lubricants that *contain* | *do not contain* hormones are the best treatment for vaginal changes due to hormone loss.
7. MAs should observe residents on hormone replacement therapy for signs and symptoms of *blood clots* | *osteoporosis*.
8. Antibiotics and fungicides should be taken *for the full amount of time they are prescribed* | *until symptoms are gone*.

4. Discuss common medications used to treat sexually transmitted infections

True or False

1. ____ Sexually transmitted infections (STIs) always have clear signs and symptoms.
2. ____ There are no medications that can cure genital herpes.
3. ____ Oral antibiotics are the most common treatment for most STIs.
4. ____ Transmission of some STIs can be reduced or stopped by using latex or polyurethane condoms.
5. ____ Antiviral medications such as acyclovir and valacyclovir can help people with syphilis stay symptom-free for longer periods of time.
6. ____ Genital HPV infection can lead to cervical cancer.
7. ____ Chlamydia, syphilis, and gonorrhea are all STIs caused by bacteria.
8. ____ Untreated STIs can cause serious complications.

19

The Immune and Lymphatic Systems and Common Medications

1. Describe the immune and lymphatic systems

Short Answer

1. What is the difference between nonspecific and specific immunity?

____

____

____

____

____

____

2. What two systems are related to the lymphatic system?

____

____

____

____

3. What are the functions of the lymphatic system?

____

____

____

____

____

____

Make a check mark (✓) next to normal changes of aging to the immune and lymphatic systems.

4. ____ Inability to recover from any kind of infection
5. ____ Increased risk of all types of infections
6. ____ Opportunistic infections occur every time a person gets sick
7. ____ It takes longer to recover from an illness
8. ____ The number and size of lymph nodes decrease
9. ____ Response to vaccines increases

2. Discuss common medications used to treat HIV/AIDS

Complete the Sentence

1. HIV affects the body in *three* | *five* stages.
2. The third stage is *chronic HIV infection* | *AIDS*.
3. HIV and AIDS destroy infection-fighting white blood cells called CD4 *thrombocytes* | *lymphocytes*.
4. The main treatment for HIV is called *antiretroviral therapy* | *radiotherapy*.
5. *Three or more* | *One or two* different drugs are used together to control HIV.
6. Pre-exposure prophylaxis is treatment given to people who *have AIDS* | *are likely to be exposed to HIV*.

7. The drugs used to treat HIV have *many* | *few* unpleasant side effects.
8. Other aspects of HIV treatment include relief of symptoms and prevention and treatment of *side effects* | *infection*.
9. It is important to observe and report signs of jaundice in residents with HIV because this could be a sign that medications are causing problems with the *liver* | *kidneys*.
10. If exposed to blood or body fluids infected with HIV, facility policy may recommend that an MA should be *put on leave* | *tested*.

3. Describe common treatments for cancer

Multiple Choice

1. What is the most likely first treatment for cancer affecting the skin, breast, colon, rectum, stomach, or muscle?
   (A) Chemotherapy
   (B) Surgery
   (C) Immunotherapy
   (D) Radiotherapy
2. Which treatment uses the person's own immune system to fight cancer?
   (A) Chemotherapy
   (B) Surgery
   (C) Immunotherapy
   (D) Radiotherapy
3. These medications given, often intravenously, to fight cancer can have severe side effects, including nausea, vomiting, diarrhea, oral sores, hair loss, fatigue, and decreased resistance to infection.
   (A) Chemotherapy
   (B) Surgery
   (C) Immunotherapy
   (D) Radiotherapy
4. This treatment destroys cells and controls cell growth in specific areas, but can also kill normal, healthy cells.
   (A) Chemotherapy
   (B) Surgery
   (C) Immunotherapy
   (D) Radiotherapy
5. Which of these medications is an MA most likely to administer to a resident with cancer?
   (A) Intravenous chemotherapy drugs
   (B) Subcutaneous injections of immunotherapy drugs
   (C) Oral antiemetic drugs
   (D) Intramuscular injections of antiemetic drugs
6. Lymphoma and leukemia are forms of cancer that primarily affect
   (A) The brain
   (B) The nerves
   (C) The gastrointestinal tract
   (D) Blood cells

Fill in the Blank

7. Cancer treatments can put residents at ______________________ risk for infection. Because of this, ______________________ infection prevention practices may be in place.
8. Cancer and cancer treatments affect each person differently. Do not make ______________________ about a resident's condition.
9. Do not apply ______________________ or any ______________________ medication to areas receiving radiation therapy unless ordered to do so.
10. Report any signs or symptoms of ______________________, such as fever, malaise, and fatigue.

4. Discuss common medications used to treat rheumatoid arthritis, lupus, and shingles

True or False

1. ____ In addition to affecting the joints, rheumatoid arthritis can affect the heart, lungs, eyes, kidneys, and skin.
2. ____ Biologic DMARDs are medications that MAs are likely to administer to residents with RA.
3. ____ NSAIDs can help slow the progress of rheumatoid arthritis.

Name: ______________________________

4. ____ Antimalarial drugs may be used to treat lupus.

5. ____ Residents with lupus who take immunosuppressants will have increased resistance to infection.

6. ____ Corticosteroids are often used to treat lupus because they slow the damaging immune response caused by the disease.

7. ____ Any person who has had chickenpox is at risk for developing shingles.

8. ____ Antiviral agents such as valacyclovir, acyclovir, and famciclovir can reduce the severity of shingles and shorten the length of the illness.

9. ____ Post-herpetic neuralgia is a form of chronic pain that occurs with lupus.

10. ____ Anticonvulsant drugs may be prescribed to reduce the pain of post-herpetic neuralgia.

11. ____ A vaccine can reduce the risk of contracting shingles.

12. ____ Shingles only affects the skin.

Name: ______________________________

Name: ______________________

Procedure Checklists

Administering oral medications			
		yes	no
1.	Identifies self by name. Identifies resident according to facility policy.		
2.	Washes hands.		
3.	Explains procedure to resident, speaking clearly, slowly, and directly. Maintains face-to-face contact whenever possible.		
4.	Provides privacy.		
5.	Puts on gloves (if required).		
6.	Raises head of bed. Makes sure resident is in an upright sitting position.		
7.	Helps resident to clean hands if she has not already done so.		
8.	Measures and documents vital signs as ordered, reporting to supervisor/holding medication as necessary.		
9.	Provides medications to resident according to preference. If both solid and liquid medications are administered, follows resident preference regarding order.		
10.	Observes as resident swallows each medication. Checks resident's mouth to make sure medication was swallowed.		
11.	Makes resident comfortable. Removes privacy measures.		
12.	Cleans and stores reusable equipment. Discards any disposable items or trash.		
13.	Removes and discards gloves if used. Washes hands.		
14.	Places call light within resident's reach.		
15.	Reports any changes in resident to nurse.		
16.	Documents administration of medication(s) on resident's MAR using facility guidelines.		

Date Reviewed	Instructor Signature
Date Performed	Instructor Signature

Name: ____________________

Administering buccal and sublingual medications		yes	no
1.	Identifies self by name. Identifies resident according to facility policy.		
2.	Washes hands.		
3.	Explains procedure to resident, speaking clearly, slowly, and directly. Maintains face-to-face contact whenever possible.		
4.	Provides privacy.		
5.	Puts on gloves (if required).		
6.	Raises head of bed. Makes sure resident is in an upright sitting position.		
7.	Helps resident to clean hands if she has not already done so.		
8.	Measures and documents vital signs as ordered, reporting to supervisor/holding medication as necessary.		
9.	Provides medication to resident. For buccal route, instructs resident to place medication between cheek and gums. For sublingual route, instructs resident to place medication under tongue. Uses gloved hands to handle and place medications (as needed).		
10.	Tells resident to allow medication to dissolve in place.		
11.	Does not leave resident's room until medication has been placed and dissolved.		
12.	Makes resident comfortable. Removes privacy measures.		
13.	Cleans and stores reusable equipment. Discards any disposable items or trash.		
14.	Removes and discards gloves if used. Washes hands.		
15.	Places call light within resident's reach.		
16.	Reports any changes in resident to nurse.		
17.	Documents administration of medication(s) on resident's MAR using facility guidelines.		

Date Reviewed ____________ Instructor Signature ____________

Date Performed ____________ Instructor Signature ____________

Name: ______________________________

Administering medications by metered dose inhaler			
		yes	no
1.	Identifies self by name. Identifies resident according to facility policy.		
2.	Washes hands.		
3.	Explains procedure to resident, speaking clearly, slowly, and directly. Maintains face-to-face contact whenever possible.		
4.	Provides privacy.		
5.	Raises head of bed. Makes sure resident is in an upright sitting position.		
6.	Measures and documents vital signs as ordered, reporting to supervisor/holding medication as necessary.		
7.	Puts on gloves (if required).		
8.	Shakes inhaler vigorously for approximately 5 seconds.		
9.	Removes cap from mouthpiece. Checks mouthpiece for any foreign object or dust.		
	If spacer is used:		
10.	Inserts inhaler mouthpiece into spacer.		
11.	Places spacer mask over nose and mouth to form a tight seal (if used). If not, asks resident to put spacer mouthpiece between teeth and lips. Holds inhaler with thumb and index finger.		
12.	Presses down firmly and quickly.		
13.	Encourages resident to breathe in slowly.		
	If spacer is not used:		
10.	Holds inhaler with thumb and index finger.		
11.	Tells resident that on count of 3 will activate inhaler. Asks resident to breathe in steadily when medication is released.		
12.	Instructs resident to breathe in and out. Places inhaler in resident's mouth.		
13.	Counts to 3. On *3*, presses inhaler down firmly and quickly and encourages resident to breathe in.		
	For both methods:		
14.	Asks resident to hold breath for 5 seconds (or as directed).		
15.	If more than one inhalation is ordered, waits approximately 1 minute before second inhalation. Shakes inhaler again before administering second inhalation.		
16.	If medication inhaled is a corticosteroid, asks resident to rinse and spit.		
17.	Replaces cap(s) on inhaler and spacer (if used).		
18.	Makes resident comfortable. Removes privacy measures.		
19.	Cleans and stores reusable equipment. Discards any disposable items or trash.		
20.	Removes and discards gloves if used. Washes hands.		
21.	Places call light within resident's reach.		
22.	Reports any changes in resident to nurse.		
23.	Documents administration of medication(s) on resident's MAR using facility guidelines.		

______________ Date Reviewed ______________ Instructor Signature

______________ Date Performed ______________ Instructor Signature

Name: ______________________________

Administering nasal medications		yes	no
1.	Identifies self by name. Identifies resident according to facility policy.		
2.	Washes hands.		
3.	Explains procedure to resident, speaking clearly, slowly, and directly. Maintains face-to-face contact whenever possible.		
4.	Provides privacy.		
5.	Puts on gloves.		
6.	Gives resident a tissue to blow nose.		
7.	Positions resident properly. If administering a nasal spray, raises head of bed. Makes sure resident is seated upright, head tilted slightly forward. If administering nasal drops, lowers head of bed with resident lying flat.		
8.	Administers medication. For nasal spray, shakes medication, then places nozzle into one nostril and squeezes to administer. Places nozzle into other nostril and squeezes to administer. For nasal drops, does not touch the dropper to nose or nostril. Allows ordered number of drops to fall into resident's nostril, toward the septum.		
9.	Encourages resident to wait at least 1 minute before wiping or blowing nose.		
10.	Makes resident comfortable. Removes privacy measures.		
11.	Cleans and stores reusable equipment. Discards any disposable items or trash.		
12.	Removes and discards gloves. Washes hands.		
13.	Places call light within resident's reach.		
14.	Reports any changes in resident to nurse.		
15.	Documents administration of medication(s) on resident's MAR using facility guidelines.		

Date Reviewed	Instructor Signature
Date Performed	Instructor Signature

Name: ___________________________________

Administering ophthalmic (eye) medications			
		yes	no
1.	Identifies self by name. Identifies resident according to facility policy.		
2.	Washes hands.		
3.	Explains procedure to resident, speaking clearly, slowly, and directly. Maintains face-to-face contact whenever possible.		
4.	Provides privacy.		
5.	Puts on gloves.		
6.	Uses a tissue to wipe resident's eye from inner canthus out. Uses a new tissue to wipe other eye if needed.		
7.	Positions resident with head tilted back (sitting upright or lying down).		
8.	Using a gloved finger, pulls lower eyelid down slightly, forming a pocket (gap) between lower lid and eye. Tells resident to look up.		
	For eye drops:		
9.	Instills a drop of medication into gap between lid and eye. Does not touch eye with dropper.		
10.	Directs resident to close eye and presses gently on inner canthus for 1 minute. Repeats as needed, waiting 5 minutes for medication to absorb before instilling second drop. Repeats with second eye if ordered.		
	For ointment:		
9.	Squeezes line of ointment into gap between eye and lower lid. Does not touch tip of tube to eyelid or eye. Repeats with second eye if ordered.		
10.	Asks resident to gently close eyes and leave them closed for several minutes.		
	For both forms:		
11.	Uses clean tissues to remove excess drops or ointment. Uses a new tissue for each eye.		
12.	Makes resident comfortable. Removes privacy measures.		
13.	Cleans and stores reusable equipment. Discards any disposable items or trash.		
14.	Removes and discards gloves. Washes hands.		
15.	Places call light within resident's reach.		
16.	Reports any changes in resident to nurse.		
17.	Documents administration of medication(s) on resident's MAR using facility guidelines.		

Date Reviewed	Instructor Signature
Date Performed	Instructor Signature

Name: ______________________

Administering otic (ear) medications

		yes	no
1.	Identifies self by name. Identifies resident according to facility policy.		
2.	Washes hands.		
3.	Explains procedure to resident, speaking clearly, slowly, and directly. Maintains face-to-face contact whenever possible.		
4.	Provides privacy.		
5.	Puts on gloves (if required).		
6.	Positions resident properly, lying down with head turned to side or seated with head tilted back and to the side.		
7.	Uses cotton ball to wipe moisture or debris from outer ear.		
8.	Straightens ear canal. Instills ordered number of drops into ear. Allows liquid to run down the side of ear canal.		
9.	Places clean cotton ball over ear canal (does not insert into ear canal). Asks resident to remain in position 3–5 minutes. Repeats with second ear if ordered.		
10.	Helps resident to a comfortable position. Removes privacy measures.		
11.	Cleans and stores reusable equipment. Discards any disposable items or trash.		
12.	Removes and discards gloves if used. Washes hands.		
13.	Places call light within resident's reach.		
14.	Reports any changes in resident to nurse.		
15.	Documents administration of medication(s) on resident's MAR using facility guidelines.		

Date Reviewed ______ Instructor Signature ______

Date Performed ______ Instructor Signature ______

Name: ______________________________

Administering topical medications

		yes	no
1.	Identifies self by name. Identifies resident according to facility policy.		
2.	Washes hands.		
3.	Explains procedure to resident, speaking clearly, slowly, and directly. Maintains face-to-face contact whenever possible.		
4.	Provides privacy.		
5.	Puts on gloves.		
6.	Positions resident properly. Exposes only body part to which medication will be applied.		
7.	Follows the medication order and manufacturer's instructions for application.		
8.	Discards used application devices.		
9.	Makes resident comfortable. Removes privacy measures.		
10.	Cleans and stores reusable equipment. Discards any disposable items or trash.		
11.	Removes and discards gloves if used. Washes hands.		
12.	Places call light within resident's reach.		
13.	Reports any changes in resident to nurse.		
14.	Documents administration of medication(s) on resident's MAR using facility guidelines.		

______________ Date Reviewed ______________ Instructor Signature

______________ Date Performed ______________ Instructor Signature

Name: ______________________

Administering warm soaks with additive			
		yes	no
1.	Identifies self by name. Identifies resident according to facility policy.		
2.	Washes hands.		
3.	Explains procedure to resident, speaking clearly, slowly, and directly. Maintains face-to-face contact whenever possible.		
4.	Provides privacy.		
5.	Puts medication or other ordered additive in basin. Fills basin half full of warm water. Follows manufacturer instructions to dissolve or mix additive. Tests water temperature with thermometer or against inside of wrist. Has resident check water temperature. Adjusts if necessary.		
6.	Places basin on a disposable absorbent pad (protective barrier) in a comfortable position for resident.		
7.	Immerses body part in basin. Pads edge of basin. Uses a bath blanket to cover resident, if needed.		
8.	Checks water temperature every 5 minutes. Adds hot water as needed. Discontinues soak if resident has pain or discomfort.		
9.	Soaks for 15 to 20 minutes or as ordered.		
10.	Removes basin. Uses towel to dry resident.		
11.	Places soiled towel in proper container.		
12.	Makes resident comfortable. Removes privacy measures.		
13.	Cleans and stores reusable equipment. Discards any disposable items or trash.		
14.	Places call light within resident's reach.		
15.	Washes hands.		
16.	Reports any changes in resident to nurse.		
17.	Documents procedure using facility guidelines. Documents administration of any medication(s) on resident's MAR.		

Date Reviewed	Instructor Signature
Date Performed	Instructor Signature

Name: ______________________________

Administering transdermal (patch) medications			
		yes	no
1.	Identifies self by name. Identifies resident according to facility policy.		
2.	Washes hands.		
3.	Explains procedure to resident, speaking clearly, slowly, and directly. Maintains face-to-face contact whenever possible.		
4.	Provides privacy.		
5.	Puts on gloves.		
6.	Positions resident properly. Exposes only body part to which medication patch will be applied.		
7.	Removes patch if one is already in place. Cleans site as directed.		
8.	Follows manufacturer instructions for discarding used transdermal medication. Does not touch patch with bare hands. Discards it so that no other person may accidentally touch it.		
9.	Removes and discards gloves. Washes hands and puts on new gloves.		
10.	Writes initials, date, and time on patch if required.		
11.	Follows medication order and manufacturer's instructions for application of new transdermal patch.		
12.	Removes and discards gloves. Washes hands.		
13.	Makes resident comfortable. Removes privacy measures.		
14.	Places call light within resident's reach.		
15.	Reports any changes in resident to nurse.		
16.	Documents administration of medication(s) on resident's MAR using facility guidelines.		

______________ Date Reviewed ______________________ Instructor Signature

______________ Date Performed ______________________ Instructor Signature

Name: ______________________

Administering a rectal suppository		yes	no
1.	Identifies self by name. Identifies resident according to facility policy.		
2.	Washes hands.		
3.	Explains procedure to resident, speaking clearly, slowly, and directly. Maintains face-to-face contact whenever possible.		
4.	Provides privacy.		
5.	Adjusts bed to safe level. Locks bed wheels.		
6.	Helps resident into left-sided Sims position. Covers with bath blanket.		
7.	Uncovers resident enough to expose buttocks only.		
8.	Unwraps suppository.		
9.	Puts on gloves.		
10.	Lubricates suppository as needed.		
11.	Spreads buttocks to expose anal area.		
12.	Uses index finger to insert suppository. Places suppository past rectal sphincter against wall of colon.		
13.	Asks resident to take deep breaths.		
14.	Withdraws finger and briefly holds toilet paper against anus. Discards toilet paper.		
15.	Removes and discards gloves. Washes hands.		
16.	Removes bath blanket and covers resident. Asks resident to retain suppository as long as possible. Makes resident comfortable.		
17.	Puts on clean gloves and provides bedpan or assistance to bathroom when needed.		
18.	Removes and discards gloves. Washes hands.		
19.	Returns bed to lowest position. Removes privacy measures.		
20.	Cleans and stores reusable equipment. Discards any disposable items or trash. Washes hands again as needed.		
21.	Places call light within resident's reach.		
22.	Reports any changes in resident to nurse.		
23.	Documents administration of medication(s) on resident's MAR using facility guidelines.		

Date Reviewed	Instructor Signature
Date Performed	Instructor Signature

Name: ______________________________

Administering medications by the vaginal route			
		yes	no
1.	Identifies self by name. Identifies resident according to facility policy.		
2.	Washes hands.		
3.	Explains procedure to resident, speaking clearly, slowly, and directly. Maintains face-to-face contact whenever possible.		
4.	Provides privacy.		
5.	Adjusts bed to safe level. Locks bed wheels.		
6.	Helps resident into dorsal recumbent position. Covers with drape.		
7.	Unwraps suppository or prepares medication applicator.		
8.	Puts on gloves.		
9.	Lubricates suppository or applicator as needed.		
10.	Inserts suppository or applicator into vagina 2–3 inches. If using an applicator, presses plunger in fully to release medication, then removes and discards applicator.		
11.	Gently wipes area around vagina with a tissue if needed. Discards tissue.		
12.	Removes and discards gloves. Washes hands.		
13.	Removes drape and covers resident.		
14.	Returns bed to lowest position. Removes privacy measures.		
15.	Places call light within resident's reach.		
16.	Reports any changes in resident to nurse.		
17.	Documents administration of medication(s) on resident's MAR using facility guidelines.		

__________ Date Reviewed ____________________ Instructor Signature

__________ Date Performed ____________________ Instructor Signature

Name: ______________________________

Practice Exam

Taking an Exam

Each state has its own rules about how medication aides become qualified to do their jobs. An exam is usually part of this process. Some states use a standardized exam called the Medication Aide Certification Exam (MACE). Others have their own state exam. You should know what the exam you will take is like. This includes knowing how many questions you will have to answer and how much time you will have. States also usually provide information on the topics covered on the exam and the number or percentage of questions to expect on each topic.

Here are some general guidelines for taking exams to help you feel better prepared:

Your physical condition affects your mental abilities. Before taking an exam, get plenty of sleep and watch what you eat and drink. On the day of the exam, eat a healthy breakfast. It can be hard to think if you are hungry or if you did not eat a nutritious breakfast. Avoid items such as energy drinks and doughnuts, which contain simple sugars.

Being in good physical shape allows for more blood to get to the brain. If you get regular physical exercise, your body uses oxygen more effectively than it would if you were out of shape. Even exercising a few days before an exam can make a noticeable difference.

When taking the exam, listen carefully to any instructions given. Be sure to read the directions and the questions carefully. If material seems unfamiliar, stay calm and reread the questions slowly. Try to eliminate answers for multiple choice questions that are clearly wrong. Your first choice is often correct, so do not change your answers unless you are sure of the correction.

Do not spend too much time on any one question. If you do not understand it, move on and go back if time and the test format allow. When you are finished with the test, review your answers if you can. Electronic tests may or may not allow you to go back to skipped questions and review answers before submission.

Remember that being nervous is natural. Most people get nervous before and during a test. A little stress can actually help you focus and make you more alert. Do not let difficult questions harm your confidence. Some questions will be challenging. Some may even cover material you have not learned or studied. This does not mean that you will not pass the exam. Taking a few deep breaths may help you calm down. Remember that the work you have chosen to do is valuable and rewarding. Try to focus on this. The exam is your chance to show that you have learned how to do this important job.

Note: There are 60 questions in this exam. The suggested time limit is 2 hours.

Practice Exam

1. An MA sees a medication listed on a resident's MAR that the MA has never administered before. What should the MA do before administering the drug for the first time?
   (A) There is no preparation needed; the MA should follow instructions on the MAR.
   (B) Ask the resident what the medication is for and follow instructions on the MAR
   (C) Read about the medication in a trusted drug reference and follow instructions on the MAR
   (D) Ask a coworker if there is anything they should know about the drug

2. When an MA enters a resident's room to administer medications, the resident's daughter is visiting. The daughter tells the MA a medication is making her mother feel dizzy. What is the best response by the MA?
   (A) The MA should report this to the nurse.
   (B) The MA should ignore this concern because it is not from the resident herself.
   (C) The MA should thank the daughter, but does not need to document or report the concern.
   (D) The MA should tell the daughter that only direct information from the resident can be considered.

3. Which of the following is true of storage for controlled medications?
   (A) They are kept in a separate building that can only be accessed by authorized staff
   (B) They are kept in double-locking storage areas
   (C) They are kept along with other medications, but must be specially marked or color coded
   (D) They are kept in a locked drawer in the room of the resident they are prescribed for

4. A drug's indications are
   (A) Cautions about possible side effects
   (B) Instructions about how it should be taken
   (C) Conditions it is approved to treat
   (D) Situations in which it should not be used

5. What is one situation in which an MA can administer a medication another person has prepared?
   (A) An MA in a state where it is allowed is assigned to administer an insulin injection prepared by the nurse
   (B) An MA is taking over a medication pass for another MA who suddenly became sick
   (C) A family member asks an MA to administer a medicinal tea he prepared at home
   (D) An MA drops a dose of a common blood pressure medication on the floor and asks another MA to "borrow" a dose from one of that MA's residents

6. Which of these is a route by which MAs may not be allowed to administer medications in all states?
   (A) Nebulization
   (B) Otic
   (C) Topical
   (D) Nasal

7. A resident has been taking a new medication for a week. Which of the following questions will give the care team the best information about the resident's experience with the new drug?
   (A) "You aren't having any side effects, are you?"
   (B) "Is that medication helping?"
   (C) "Tell me how you've been feeling since you started the new medication."
   (D) "Do you think you want to stick with that new medication?"

8. After frequent resident complaints at an LTCF that medications are not controlling their pain, it is discovered that a healthcare worker has been replacing strong painkillers with stock acetaminophen and taking the painkillers to sell. This crime is called
   (A) Substitution
   (B) Negligence
   (C) Diversion
   (D) Distraction

9. Which types of medications should be stored in separate areas?
   (A) Oral medications and sublingual or buccal medications
   (B) Short-acting and long-acting bronchodilators
   (C) Oral medications and topical medications
   (D) Rectal suppositories and vaginal suppositories

10. An MA has just administered acetaminophen, with the nurse's approval, to a resident who has a PRN order for the drug to relieve arthritis pain. After administering the drug the MA realizes she has administered the wrong strength: two 500-mg tablets instead of the two 350-mg tablets indicated on the resident's MAR. Which of the following is true?
    (A) Because an OTC medication is involved, this is not considered a medication error
    (B) This is a medication error, but because it involves an OTC medication, it does not need to be reported or documented.
    (C) This is a medication error, but it is unlikely to harm the resident; to avoid getting in trouble, the MA should not mention it.
    (D) This is a medication error and must be reported and documented according to facility policy.

11. Providers able to order medications include
    (A) Vocational nurses, registered nurses, and physicians
    (B) Registered nurses, physician assistants, and physicians
    (C) Nurse practitioners, physician assistants, and physicians
    (D) Charge nurses, medical directors, and directors of nursing

12. When an authorized healthcare professional receives a verbal (oral) medication order, what must be done immediately?
    (A) It must be put in writing and read back to confirm that it is correct.
    (B) The first dose must be administered and then the order put in writing.
    (C) The provider must send a fax confirming the order.
    (D) A physician on-site must agree that the order is appropriate.

13. A complete medication order includes
    (A) Brand name, dose, and physical description (e.g., a round, blue scored tablet)
    (B) Brand or generic name, strength, form, dose, directions, and refills
    (C) Generic name, physical description, timing of administration, and side effects
    (D) Brand name, dose, form, expected cost, and refills

14. Medications in spray form are most commonly administered by these routes:
    (A) Nasal, topical, sublingual
    (B) Inhalation, nebulization, oral
    (C) Topical, ophthalmic, otic
    (D) Optic, otic, topical

15. When should an MA document that a medication has been administered?
    (A) During the third medication safety check
    (B) When the medication is removed from storage
    (C) When the package is replaced in storage
    (D) After the resident has taken the medication

16. What may need to be documented in addition to the fact that a medication was administered?
    (A) Whether the resident had family visiting at the time
    (B) Vital sign measurements taken before a medication was administered
    (C) The amount of food the resident ate at the previous meal
    (D) The resident's general mood

17. Which of the following is an analgesic?
    (A) Salmeterol/fluticasone
    (B) Hydrocodone/acetaminophen
    (C) Amoxicillin/clavulanate
    (D) Betamethasone/clotrimazole

Name: ______________________________

18. An MA is most likely to be allowed to dispose of
    (A) A single dose of medication that falls on the floor before it can be administered
    (B) A full package of medication that a resident no longer needs
    (C) Any amount of medication that remains after a resident has died
    (D) Any amount of medication that is a controlled substance

19. An MA is about to administer medications and asks a resident to state their full name and date of birth. The resident says, "Marietta, February 19." Has the MA successfully checked for *right resident*?
    (A) Yes. The resident has provided name and date of birth.
    (B) Possibly, if the MA knows this resident well and recognizes that it is the correct resident
    (C) No. The resident gave her date of birth correctly, but did not give her full name.
    (D) No. The resident did not give her full name or her full date of birth.

20. The difference between a medication that is administered by the *otic route* and a medication that is administered by the *optic route* is
    (A) Medications administered by the otic route are placed in the ear and medications administered by the optic route are placed in the eye
    (B) Medications administered by the otic route are placed in the eye and medications administered by the optic route are placed in the ear
    (C) Medications administered by the otic route are placed in the nose and medications administered by the optic route are placed in the eye
    (D) Not significant; they are different ways of spelling the same route of administration

21. Which of the following is determined by law?
    (A) How a facility organizes medication setup and medication passes
    (B) The minimum number of hours a part-time MA can work
    (C) The length and type of training an MA must have
    (D) The maximum number of medications a resident can take

22. A resident's full name and date of birth must be checked against
    (A) The MAR and the medication label when a drug is administered for the first time
    (B) The MAR and the medication label every time a drug is administered
    (C) Either the MAR or the medication label every time a drug is administered
    (D) The MAR and the resident's room number every time a drug is administered

23. A resident has a PRN order for 700 mg of acetaminophen up to three times a day for headache. A nurse has assessed the resident and approved administration of the medication. To administer the right dose, an MA must check
    (A) How many tablets are in the bottle
    (B) The strength of the tablets in the bottle
    (C) How many tablets the resident wants to take
    (D) The size of the tablets in the bottle

24. If a resident does not want to take a medication, what must be documented?
    (A) How the MA convinced the resident to take the medication anyway
    (B) That the medication was refused
    (C) Whether the MA agrees with the resident's reason for refusal
    (D) Whether the resident is generally challenging to work with

25. Knowing if a medication must be administered before, with, or after a meal is part of administering the medication
    (A) To the right resident
    (B) At the right dose
    (C) By the right route
    (D) At the right time

26. If an MA works in a state that allows MAs to split medications (as ordered), which of these medications may be split?
    (A) Any tablet
    (B) Only tablets with an enteric coating
    (C) Only tablets without a coating
    (D) Only scored tablets

27. A bottle of over-the-counter liquid cold and flu medication contains 360 mL of liquid. The active ingredients are acetaminophen and phenylephrine. Which of the following describes the *strength* of the medication?
    (A) There are 360 mL of liquid in the bottle.
    (B) There are 12 doses in the bottle.
    (C) There are 325 mg of acetaminophen and 5 mg of phenylephrine in each 15 mL of liquid.
    (D) There are 2 active ingredients in the medication.

28. What is the most common route of medication administration?
    (A) Oral
    (B) Ophthalmic
    (C) Injection
    (D) Inhalation

29. An MA enters a resident's room as the resident is having a telehealth visit with his provider. When she sees the MA, the provider says, "I want you to increase Mr. Tien's lisinopril dose to 15 mg." Which of the following is the best response?
    (A) "Yes, ma'am. I will get that changed in the MAR right away."
    (B) "Can you repeat that, please? I want to write it down. Then I will repeat it back to you before I change it in the MAR."
    (C) "I already have his 10-mg dose ready for today. Is it OK if we start this tomorrow?"
    (D) "I'm sorry, but I can't take a medication order. If you give me a minute I can get my supervisor."

30. Medications in suppository form are administered by
    (A) The rectal or vaginal route
    (B) The sublingual or buccal route
    (C) The oral or rectal route
    (D) The subcutaneous or intravenous route

31. When checking for *right medication,* MAs should pay very close attention to tall man lettering because it is used
    (A) To emphasize the brand name of a drug
    (B) To mark drugs that are considered controlled substances
    (C) To mark drugs with names that may be confused with other drug names
    (D) To mark drugs that have boxed warnings

32. One of the most significant factors that affects how the body uses medication and must be considered in drug dosing is
    (A) Length of illness
    (B) Exercise habits
    (C) Age
    (D) Attitude toward taking medications

33. Body composition refers to
    (A) How tall a person is
    (B) Whether a person is male or female
    (C) A person's physical traits such as hair and eye color
    (D) The amount of muscular tissue and fatty tissue in the body

34. What is the difference between an oral disintegrating tablet and a sublingual tablet?
    (A) An oral disintegrating tablet is chewed and a sublingual tablet is allowed to dissolve.
    (B) An oral disintegrating tablet is swallowed with water and a sublingual tablet is allowed to dissolve in the mouth.
    (C) An oral disintegrating tablet is stirred into a cup of liquid and a sublingual tablet is allowed to dissolve under the tongue.
    (D) An oral disintegrating tablet is allowed to dissolve in the mouth and a sublingual tablet is allowed to dissolve under the tongue.

35. At a minimum, how many times should an MA check a medication against the MAR before administering it to a resident?
    (A) 1 time
    (B) 2 times
    (C) 3 times
    (D) 4 times

36. Which of the following lists of medications is likely to be on the MAR of a resident who has coronary artery disease?
    (A) Atorvastatin, lisinopril, aspirin, and nitroglycerin
    (B) Fluticasone, albuterol, and prednisone
    (C) Metformin, sitagliptin, and insulin
    (D) Carbidopa/levodopa and benztropine

37. Where would an MA learn that a boxed warning applies to a particular drug?
    (A) On the resident's MAR and on the outer packaging of the drug
    (B) In the facility's policy manual and on a drug inventory list
    (C) In a drug reference resource and the drug's package insert
    (D) In eMAR software and in the resident's chart

38. These classes of medications can increase bleeding risk:
    (A) Antidepressants, antibiotics, and antitussives
    (B) Anticoagulants, antiplatelet agents, and NSAIDs
    (C) Bile acid sequestrants, statins, and fibrates
    (D) Antacids, proton pump inhibitors, and H2 blockers

39. Which of the following is true about whether to write *2.0 mL* or *2 mL* when referring to medication doses?
    (A) Writing *2.0 mL* is correct because it is standard scientific form.
    (B) Writing *2.0 mL* is correct because it is more precise.
    (C) Writing *2 mL* is correct because it takes less time.
    (D) Writing *2 mL* is correct because it cannot be mistaken for *20 mL*.

40. Two residents at a facility have the same name, Jennifer Green. How can an MA ensure medications are administered to the right resident?
    (A) By suggesting that one of the residents should go by *Jenny*
    (B) By asking each resident to state full name and date of birth and checking this against the MAR and medication label every time medications are administered
    (C) By asking each resident to confirm the names of the medications she takes each time medications are administered
    (D) By keeping a list of each resident's medications on the resident's bedside table

41. An MA has been administering an antibiotic to a resident 3 times a day for 3 days. When the MA brings the medication in on the morning of the fourth day, the resident says, "That medicine is giving me diarrhea and I feel better anyway. I'll take it if I have to, but could I just stop?" Which of the following should the MA do?
    (A) Hold the medication and document that the resident has diarrhea
    (B) Hold the medication and tell the resident to let her know the next time she comes by if the diarrhea has stopped
    (C) Tell the resident that she should continue taking the medication and assure her the diarrhea will go away soon
    (D) Tell the resident that she should continue taking the medication and document and report resident's diarrhea

42. Which of the following tasks may be delegated to an MA?
    (A) Inserting a feeding tube to administer a medication to a resident who cannot have anything by mouth
    (B) Adjusting the amount of warfarin administered based on results of a fingerstick test of blood clotting time
    (C) Deciding when to administer a PRN over-the-counter medication
    (D) Measuring vital signs before administering certain drugs

43. If a resident whose blood pressure is normally close to 120/80 has a blood pressure reading of 104/65, what should an MA do?
   (A) Nothing. This reading is in normal range.
   (B) Report to the nurse. This reading is different from the resident's baseline.
   (C) Hold any blood pressure medications on the resident's MAR.
   (D) Suggest that the resident add extra salt to his food to bring his blood pressure up a bit.

44. Furosemide (Lasix) is a common medication. Residents who take furosemide may need to
   (A) Limit strenuous exercise
   (B) Use the bathroom often
   (C) Limit their consumption of green leafy vegetables
   (D) Stay out of direct sunlight and/or wear protective clothing

45. When taking oral medications, a resident should be in this position:
   (A) Supine
   (B) Semi-Fowler (30–45 degrees)
   (C) Fowler (45–60 degrees)
   (D) Upright (90 degrees)

46. Which of these groups of foods have known interactions with medications?
   (A) Grapefruit, dairy, leafy greens
   (B) Apples, whole grains, and legumes
   (C) Eggs, hard cheeses, and melon
   (D) Nut butters, bread products, and apple juice

47. After taking a medication that was prescribed to help him relax and sleep, a resident reports that he was awake and anxious most of the night. This may be an example of
   (A) Idiosyncratic reaction
   (B) Anaphylactic reaction
   (C) Systemic reaction
   (D) Paradoxical reaction

48. A resident who has taken penicillin before with no adverse reaction develops hives and has difficulty breathing half an hour after taking penicillin. This reaction
   (A) May be anaphylaxis and must have been triggered by something other than the penicillin
   (B) May be anaphylaxis and may have been triggered by the penicillin
   (C) Cannot be anaphylaxis because the resident has taken penicillin before
   (D) Cannot be anaphylaxis because hives and difficulty breathing are not symptoms of anaphylaxis

49. Which of the following types of medications must be primed before first use?
   (A) Buccal films and oral disintegrating tablets
   (B) Nasal sprays and metered dose inhalers
   (C) Eye ointment tubes and ear drops
   (D) Nebulized medications and oxygen

50. A resident who takes levothyroxine to treat hypothyroidism will usually have the medication administered
   (A) An hour before breakfast or right before bedtime
   (B) Three times a day with meals
   (C) 30–60 minutes after breakfast
   (D) With the evening meal

51. An MA is outside a resident's room preparing medications at a cart. A nursing assistant asks the MA to help her transfer a resident. Which of the following is the best response from the MA?
   (A) Look up and say, "Give me a minute. I have to finish setting up these meds first."
   (B) Look up and say, "OK. But we'll have to be quick so I don't forget where I was."
   (C) Keep focusing on the medications and, when she is at a stopping point, say, "I'm sorry, but I'm doing a medication pass and can't help right now."
   (D) Keep focusing on the medications and, when she is at a stopping point, shout, "Leave me alone! I'm setting up meds!"

Name: ______________________

52. What is an MA likely to be required to do before administering digoxin to a resident?
   (A) Weigh the resident
   (B) Measure the resident's blood pressure
   (C) Count the resident's apical pulse rate
   (D) Count the resident's respirations

53. A resident has an order for both eye drops and ointment to be administered in the same eye. Unless the medication instructions say otherwise, how should the MA administer them?
   (A) Administer the ointment first. Wait 5 minutes. Administer the eye drops.
   (B) Administer the ointment first. Administer the eye drops immediately after.
   (C) Administer the eye drops first. Wait 5 minutes. Administer the ointment.
   (D) Administer the eye drops first. Administer the ointment immediately after.

54. When the action of one drug decreases or cancels the effects of another drug, the interaction is called
   (A) Addition
   (B) Synergism
   (C) Potentiation
   (D) Antagonism

55. The abbreviations *b.i.d.* and *t.i.d.* relate to
   (A) The number of times per day a drug should be administered
   (B) The route by which a drug should be administered
   (C) The time of day at which a drug should be administered
   (D) Vital sign measurements

56. Which of these pairs of residents is most likely to have different responses to the same dose of the same drug?
   (A) A 90-year-old female who weighs 120 pounds and an 85-year-old female who weighs 130 pounds
   (B) An 82-year-old male who weighs 145 pounds and a 78-year-old male who weighs 160 pounds
   (C) An 88-year-old female and a 70-year-old female who both weigh 155 pounds
   (D) A 72-year-old male who weighs 220 pounds and a 95-year-old female who weighs 105 pounds

57. A resident's MAR lists a medication to be administered at a dose of 100 mg. An MA setting up medications for the resident sees that the medication was dispensed by the pharmacy as 200-mg tablets. What should the MA do?
   (A) Use a pill splitter to cut a tablet in half
   (B) Correct the MAR to read 200 mg
   (C) Administer the medication and then report the situation to the nurse
   (D) Do not administer the medication and report the situation to the nurse

58. Beta-blockers, ARBs, and ACE inhibitors are all
   (A) Antihypertensive drugs
   (B) Antihyperlipidemic drugs
   (C) Antispasmodic drugs
   (D) Anxiolytic drugs

59. Most medications should be stored
   (A) In a refrigerator kept between 35°F and 40°F
   (B) In a freezer kept close to 0°F
   (C) In an area kept at high humidity and a temperature of at least 75°F
   (D) In a dry area protected from sunlight at a comfortable room temperature

60. Which of the following is true of proton pump inhibitors?
    (A) Used to treat hypertension; names end in *-olol;* blood pressure may be measured before administration
    (B) Used to treat high cholesterol; names end in *-statin;* often administered at bedtime
    (C) Used to treat GERD; names end in *-prazole;* should be administered 30–60 minutes before a meal
    (D) Used to treat GERD; names end in *-tidine;* decrease acid production

Name: ___________________________

Name: ______________________________

Name: ______________________________